"This book provides an excellent conceptualization of engaging and adapting traditional family therapy models for neurodiverse individuals and their families. Excellent case examples and relevant applications of techniques are provided that are likely to be helpful for clients and clinicians alike."

Eric Mitchell, PhD, *owner and director of Neurodiversity Consultants LLC*

"This book is a must-read for anyone working with individuals on the autism spectrum and their families. The authors create a primer for mastering sociocultural domain effects for this group. As a child psychiatrist and parent of an adult living with autism, I found this groundbreaking book to resonate with empathy and passion for patient care."

Mike Colston, MD, *Captain (retired) US Navy*

"*Treating Families on the Spectrum* provides a systemic lens and useful clinical tools. Even experienced therapists will gain new insights and perspectives that can help families navigate the complex, challenging, and nuanced differences that autism presents."

Robert Naseef, PhD, *psychologist, author, parent of adult autistic child*

Treating Families on the Spectrum

This book outlines how therapists and families who have a child with autism spectrum disorder (ASD) can use an ecological systems approach, which offers a holistic and nuanced model that treats the entire family system rather than just the individual.

Filled with case studies and empirically supported suggestions from clinical practice, this comprehensive book provides an applied therapeutic model that supports the whole family, highlighting how various levels of autism can present differing challenges from a family systems lens. Written using a lifespan developmental framework, chapters begin with early diagnosis and cover essential milestones from childhood to adulthood, addressing issues such as clinical concerns for families, children in school, the role of siblings, the extended family, the assessment process, and the anticipated loss of caregivers. This essential resource aims to not reduce behavioral concerns of autism but rather strengthen the entire family system. Going beyond psychoeducation, this book provides practical and clinical approaches to helping families navigate the unique challenges and family dynamics of autism.

This book is designed to be read by mental health professionals such as social workers, psychologists, psychiatrists, and marriage and family therapists, as well as family members themselves.

Britney Fontes, PsyD, is a clinical psychologist at a state psychiatric hospital in New Jersey. She graduated from Chestnut Hill College in Philadelphia. She has been noted as a behavioral and psychodynamic therapist who works primarily with individuals who have serious, persistent mental illnesses and developmental disabilities.

Gwendolyn Edwards, PsyD, is a clinical psychologist at a medical hospital in Lewisburg, Pennsylvania. She graduated from Chestnut Hill College in Philadelphia. She has been noted as a systemic and psychodynamic therapist who works primarily with individuals and families with various mental health disorders.

Scott Browning, PhD, ABPP, is Professor Emeritus of psychology in the doctoral program at Chestnut Hill College. He is a widely published author of *The Contemporary Family, Translating Research into Practice,* and *Stepfamily Therapy.* Scott Browning has received awards from the American Psychological Association and the Pennsylvania Psychological Association for his contribution to Family Psychology.

Treating Families on the Spectrum

An Ecological Systems Approach

Britney Fontes, Gwendolyn Edwards, and Scott Browning

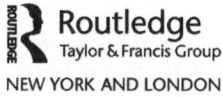
Routledge
Taylor & Francis Group

NEW YORK AND LONDON

Designed cover image: Getty Images

First published 2025
by Routledge
605 Third Avenue, New York, NY 10158

and by Routledge
4 Park Square, Milton Park, Abingdon, Oxon, OX14 4RN

Routledge is an imprint of the Taylor & Francis Group, an informa business

ISBN: 978-1-032-58734-9 (hbk)
ISBN: 978-1-032-58733-2 (pbk)
ISBN: 978-1-003-45126-6 (ebk)

DOI: 10.4324/9781003451266

Typeset in Sabon
by Newgen Publishing UK

To my incredible friends and family who have supported me throughout this journey of pursuing my dream to become an author, especially to my amazing mother, Lori Fontes. But most importantly, to the families of autism who inspired me to write this book. Thank you for allowing me into your world; without your honesty and love, this book would not be possible.

– Britney Fontes

To Owen, who taught me how to be a member of a family on the autism spectrum.

– Scott Browning

To the remarkable individuals I've had the privilege to work with, whose courage and perseverance inspire every page, and to my family whose unwavering support has fueled this journey—this book is a tribute to the power of understanding and love in navigating autism spectrum disorder.

– Gwendolyn Edwards

Contents

Introduction

If you are a parent, clinician, teacher, provider, a family member of a person on the spectrum, a student, or just someone who wants to better understand how to treat autism, you are in the right place. This book was inspired by the complex and unique experiences of families on the spectrum and our love for family therapy through a systemic approach. A family system is made up of individual parts. Each person represents one of those essential parts. Each person in a family will bring various personalities, strengths, limitations, and experiences that create the culture of that family dynamic. Some family dynamics and emotional environments are well-oiled machines that engage with one another with ease, though, as many know, most families will experience some degree of stress, conflict, tragedy, or road bumps that can put any strong family to the test. This is true whether someone in a family has autism or not. A person with autism exists in a layered system of other parts. Thus, we propose that a person with autism cannot be treated or supported in isolation. As authors and experts in the field of treating families through various evidence-supported and evidence-based treatments, we are not suggesting that all families with autism will struggle. Research supports that many families of autism are not worse off than neurotypical families but rather create their own sense of normalcy. In short, being part of a family with autism is just different. Many families with autism may even function as though autism does not exist at all. However, we intend to highlight real-life challenges that many families may encounter over the span of one's life. We also aspire to provide guidance to even the strongest of families. We acknowledge that this book might be read by parents, clinicians, students, physicians, teachers, or simply someone who is passionate about family systems or autism. One does not need to be related to or know someone with autism to benefit from reading this book. We discuss family phenomena that can be applied to most families because the foundations and concepts of the ecological systems approach are consistent regardless of family makeup. We encourage individuals who do not have personal connections with autism to challenge themselves to think critically about how family system concepts can relate to their own family dynamics or that of the population they are most interested in. This book will follow several clinical case examples that cover various levels of autism, different stages of development, common challenges, and how families can address these concerns in therapy. The case examples also provide real clinical interventions that professionals and clinicians can utilize. Families may use the clinical cases as guides to address certain concerns in their own lives with various disciplines. We explore case examples that describe how families can face realistic academic, therapeutic, and family challenges. An important feature of this book that has historically been missing in the literature is that it highlights the concerns of older adults on the spectrum. We hope to provide families and clinicians with essential psychoeducation about special services and the challenges families may need to process, such as crises, residential placements, and finances. This book will cover diagnosis, the Autism Trait Scale (ATS), cultural intersections, assessment evaluations, individualized educational programs, public versus private settings, individual rights of students, siblings impacts, the inclusion of extended family, the aging adult on the spectrum, and common challenges families may experience.

1 The Basics

"What you need to know" about Autism and Diversity

Britney Fontes

What Is Autism?

Autism is a neurodevelopmental disorder that presents on a spectrum of persistent impairments in social communication and social interactions as well as restricted or repetitive patterns of behavior or interests and activities (5th ed.; DSM-5; American Psychiatric Association, 2013). In order for a person to be diagnosed with autism, they must experience the symptoms stated above during early childhood, and symptoms must impair or limit daily functioning. If a person is seeking an autism diagnosis, they should seek a formal psychoeducational or psychological assessment through a school, a licensed mental health professional, or a licensed psychologist. One person with autism may look very different from the next person with autism, reflecting the true spectrum in which a person can fall any-where on a continuum. An individual who is diagnosed with autism at age five years old may have significant delays in verbal communication, severe sensitivity to certain sounds and textures, may struggle with transitions, demonstrate dysregulation of mood, and may spend hours every day organizing their matchbox cars by color. This child may begin school being behind in reading and math, as well as appear much younger than their chronological age compared to their peers. Another person with autism may get a diagnosis much later in life, at the age of 16 years old, have few friends, demonstrate stimming behaviors when upset or excited but can mask these when around others, be placed in advanced academic classes, be able to share any and all facts about the president, and may be on an accelerated route to graduating high school early to pursue a law degree. These examples demonstrate classic examples of the differences in the degree of functioning, skills, and life trajectories of a person on the autism spectrum. Of course, these are only two examples of the endless presentations of autism.

DOI: 10.4324/9781003451266-1

Identity Language

The language around autism continues to change. There was a time when embracing the term "autistic" was seen as the proper way to recognize that one cannot take medication and no longer be autistic. Then, people moved to using the term "person with autism" to recognize the diagnosis but highlight the person first. More recently, the term "neurodiverse," as in "neurodiverse child," has become preferred to highlight that the neurodiverse community is, in fact, diverse and a culture unto itself. The authors of this book agree strongly with the recognition of autism as forming a culture. However, regarding language, this book continues with the person-first language. It should be noted that how a family or person wants to identify or use specific language, such as autistic person, neurodiverse child, a person diagnosed with autism, neurodivergent, a person with autism, and so on, is indeed a preference. There is no right or wrong answer regarding the language or identities previously listed, thus highlighting the true essence of culture, in that a person gets to choose how they define themselves, especially when it comes to identity language. The authors encourage clinicians and providers to ask families what identity language they prefer and what feels most inclusive or salient to them. Similarly, families should communicate their preferences. Another term also commonly associated with autism due to its nature of being on a spectrum is "low/high functioning." Although there are not necessarily new ways to describe the spectrum of autism, for some, these terms can be controversial and are not perfect by any means. However, for consistency and to provide a teaching model that describes levels of autism in various domains of functioning, the authors will use low/medium/high functioning terminology throughout the book.

Does a person with Autism always have Autism?

The answer to the question above is yes. A person with autism may begin to experience difficulties by the second year of life, but it is possible to see signs earlier than 12 months. There is no cure for autism because it is a neurodevelopmental disorder, meaning there is a reasonably strong genetic component that is responsible for autism spectrum disorder (ASD), essentially affecting one's brain development. In short, the autistic brain is different. Since there is limited research that examines the neuropathology and neuroimaging of autistic brains, there is little evidence of biological autism advances. However, it is worth noting that some studies suggest potential abnormalities in early brain development, such as brain overgrowth (Geschwind, 2008). Although there are no specific identifications in neurobiological mechanisms at this time (National Research Council

(2001), a person's genetic heritability can range anywhere from 37% to 90% (5th ed.; DSM-5; American Psychiatric Association, 2013). Many risk factors can increase a person's likelihood of having autism, regardless of their rate of genetic heritability. For example, the environment proposes several risk factors, including advanced maternal age, low birth weight, or fetal exposure to certain medications used for mental health or medical concerns. To be clear, if someone gives birth to a child at an older age, that does not mean their child will automatically have autism; it simply means that the percentage and chance of risk increase.

Can Autism Share Similar Symptoms with Other Diagnoses?

Yes, while autism is vastly unique and different in each person, it can often share similar symptoms with other diagnoses. For example, autism features can overlap or appear as an intellectual disability, as global developmental delay, a language disorder, a social pragmatic or unspecified communication disorder, as Rett syndrome, as selective mutism, as attention deficit hyperactive disorder (ADHD), or as schizophrenia (5th ed.; DSM-5; American Psychiatric Association, 2013). Not only can symptoms overlap, but a person with autism can also have a comorbid diagnosis that resembles varying degrees of symptoms and challenges. In other words, a person can have both autism and an intellectual impairment or language disorder, which are common for people on the spectrum. The Centers for Disease Control and Prevention (CDC) found that in 2016, 33% of children eight years old also met the criteria for an intellectual disability, meaning their intelligence quotient (IQ) was below 70. Of this population, girls were 6% more likely to meet the criterion of an intellectual disability than boys. Interestingly, and more recently, the *Diagnostic and Statistical Manual of Mental Disorders* (DSM) edited their diagnostic criteria for autism. The current diagnostic manual has removed specific categories within autism, such as autistic disorder, pervasive developmental disorder not otherwise specified, and Asperger's syndrome (America Psychiatric Association, 2013). The *DSM-5* has shifted to a broader and more inclusive description that focuses on the severity of symptoms, also known as levels, while also reducing the number of symptoms required in each domain and combining domains, such as communication and social behavior. One can assume that as time passes, the description of autism will continue to evolve. Grzadzinski, Huerta, and Lord (2013) explored the potential benefits of the updated *DSM-5* and its impacts on research through understanding autism on a spectrum rather than what has typically been utilized as exclusive subtypes. Grzadzinski and colleagues explain that by expanding *DSM* criteria, researchers can obtain larger, more homogeneous sample sizes, resulting in a more accurate interpretation of the data and the likelihood that others can replicate studies. Essentially, by looking at autism on a spectrum with broader criteria, one can study and better understand more individuals.

Who has Autism?

The CDC has estimated that 1 in 36 children eight years old have autism (2020). These results were found by examining data collected by the Autism and Developmental Disabilities Monitoring (ADDM) Network, which is an active surveillance program that keeps track of autism estimates across 11 sites in the United States. These estimates are reliable because each autism diagnosis was confirmed by medical health professionals and not simply by parental reports or by guessing that a child has autism. Interestingly, in 2014, the CDC found that about 1 in 68 children in the United States had an ASD diagnosis, which results in about a 32% increase in prevalence rates since the most recent review. It may be the case that when this book is published, there will be more children diagnosed with autism who have yet to be documented, influencing overall prevalence rates. There may be several reasons why the prevalence of autism appears to be increasing. One reason could be due to advancements in research and a better, more holistic understanding of autism, which allows medical and mental health providers to diagnose autism at an earlier age. Another reason could be that diagnostic criteria are expanding to encompass a full spectrum of symptoms and challenges, thus allowing for a more reliable and accurate diagnosis. In other words, instead of clinicians being puzzled whether a child may have what was once known as a developmental disorder not otherwise specified or Asperger's syndrome, they can accurately identify a person on the autism spectrum.

Diversity in Autism

Before you continue to read, take a moment to reflect on the possible prevalence of autism among different ethnoracial groups. Take a guess as to how often you believe specific groups may get diagnosed compared to others. The CDC (2016) found that eight-year-olds who identify as White, Black, and Asian/Pacific Islander had nearly identical rates of autism. However, Hispanic children had significantly lower rates of an autism diagnosis. Researchers in Georgia examined educational mechanisms, criteria, methods used in public school systems and found that students from ethnically diverse backgrounds were less likely to be identified, whereas their white counterparts were overrepresented (Morrier et al., 2008). The researchers propose that one reason children who are ethnically diverse may be underrepresented could be due to the lack of information and access to resources provided to families, especially at a young age. It is essential that information about early indicators be readily available and provided by professionals who serve ethnically diverse groups. Interestingly, Morrier and colleagues also found that the majority of teachers in the public school system in Georgia who provide educational services for autism are majority white, which presents a cultural mismatch for ethnically diverse students. A cultural mismatch, meaning two people having different cultural identities, such as students and their teachers, can consequently lead school faculty to assign children to more restrictive placements (Hops & Reschly, 2003; Morrier et al., 2008). One fascinating literature review explored the diversity within multiethnic and multilingual families who receive autism treatment, such as applied behavior analysis (ABA) (Wang et al., 2019). The researchers make a valuable point that ethnoracial families face more challenges in the United States when their child gets diagnosed with autism. For example, there are fewer trained ABA therapists who speak multiple languages, such as the native languages of many ethnically diverse families. ABA therapists may also lack cultural awareness of the multiethnic families they could treat, thus limiting families from seeking support. Wang et al. (2019) also discuss the financial burdens that families may face raising a child on the spectrum. More importantly, the reality is that families have difficulty obtaining reliable healthcare if they have a child who was born outside of the United States. This may result in family members quitting their jobs to take care of their child with autism full-time, further exacerbating financial burdens and access to assessment and treatment (Sen & Yurtsever, 2007). As we think about culture, let us reflect on the vast values, beliefs, and practices that encompass an individual on a small and a large scale. Some groups may share similar traditions within their cultural group but still may have unique practices with their close family. One would expect that our cultural beliefs influence how we seek treatment, experience support, make sense of mental health diagnoses, and utilize and have access to family support, as well as general quality of life. Some groups may not have the terminology or an understanding of autism due to differences in cultural perception and vocabulary, thus creating another obstacle in receiving early support and diagnosis of autism. Sen and Yurtsever (2007) go so far as to propose that what may be seen in one culture as a symptom or problem can be appropriate or accepted in another. In other words, ideas about autism and how one treats autism are filtered through a Westernized cultural lens, thus biasing what one believes as problematic. More specifically, take a moment to consider how different cultures communicate and express emotions, thoughts, and behaviors. Wang et al. (2019) discuss the essential point that some cultures have different social norms. For example, in Asian cultures, children are often taught from a young age to avoid eye contact with adults and limit facial expressions (Kitzhaber, 2012; Wang et al., 2019). Avoiding eye contact and restricted facial expressions may overlap or reflect symptoms of autism. However, if a child is presenting as such, they may be overlooked as expressing typical nonverbal behavior within their cultural context when, in fact, these could be signs of autism, resulting in a later diagnosis compared to white children. Another example is the differences in social behaviors across cultures that may not be appropriate for ABA treatment of autism. For example, the degree to which we use eye contact, personal space, movement of the body, or volume and tone of voice may vastly shift from one family to the next. ABA treatment often falls short by not considering cultural norms and values that conflict with actual progression and social comfort outside of autism. For example, lack of eye contact may be culturally motivated rather than reflect a lack of social understanding or social communication deficit. An ABA therapist would need to be culturally informed to work on social communication and behavior while also respecting diversity and what is appropriate within each family. In some cultures, a child should not greet adults in the same way they greet other children or peers. An ABA therapist may misinterpret this interaction as a lack of skills, or encourage the child with autism to interact differently with elders, thus creating a cultural rupture within the family treatment and missing the opportunity for contextually informed interventions. It appears that some ethnically diverse families are underrepresented in the diagnosis and treatment of autism while also not receiving equal and accessible care. This fact alone creates a crisis for families who are not valued or seen in similar ways as families from Caucasian backgrounds.

Gender...Let's Talk About It

Boys are four and a half times more likely to be diagnosed with autism than girls. Specifically, the estimated ASD prevalence was 23.4 per 1,000 boys (one in 43 boys) and 5.2 per 1,000 girls (one in 193 girls) (Christensen et al., 2016). This finding is not surprising because, historically, boys have been disproportionately diagnosed with autism. Why might this happen? First, it is important to note that traditionally, research about autism has included more males in studies. This bias may result in testing materials and instruments being better at identifying autism in males. It may also be the case that females express autism symptoms in different ways compared to males, which implies they would meet the criteria for an autism diagnosis in diverse ways. For example, some females are better at expressing behaviors, such as reciprocal communication and adjusting their behavior to the situation (Lai et al., 2015). This occurrence may be due to Westernized culture, which socializes females from an early age to take on gender role expectations, resulting in more interpersonal processes. Girls are often subconsciously raised to appear "submissive and respectful," following specific social scripts, which also influence how autism symptoms may appear in different stages of development. Lai and colleagues (2015) also explored bias in how professionals interpret autism in females, such as seeing the personality trait of being shy as typical for girls, or misdiagnosing ASD symptoms as anxiety or depression.

For example, let us think about observing children in a classroom. Imagine an eight-year-old girl sitting on the floor in the book circle by herself. The girl is quietly reading and enjoying a book about birds, seemingly unphased by the children around her. Another child approaches the girl and asks if she would like to help them build a house out of blocks, but the girl shakes her head and says, "That is OK. I am reading, thank you." Another child approaches and asks if he can look at the book with her. The girl replies, "I am not done yet, but you can have it after." What is happening appears to be a quiet young girl having socially appropriate interactions with her peers. Her interpersonal abilities appear typical, and if anything, she may just be shy and like to spend time alone. What one might overlook is that this girl only reads books about birds or that during her free time, she only spends it by herself and will become distressed when someone is sitting too close to her. Although she knows in school, you "play nice with others," and it is more expected that she follow the social script, so she rarely tells other children to move away from her. This is also known as masking, which many people with autism may do to hide their internal emotional distress. If we imagined this example with a boy who only reads books about dinosaurs and likes to be alone, but will more often tell other kids to move away from him or tell children bluntly, "No, I don't like building houses," there is a chance the boy will more likely be evaluated for autism than the girl. You may be thinking, well, sure, the boy responded differently than the girl. However, this is partly the problem with misinterpretation. How we interpret symptoms is biased by gender role expectations. We may expect a girl to be polite, so her presentation should not be concerning, whereas we may tolerate boys being more expressive and direct than girls. Still, in doing so, the boy's behavior may grab our attention first. Both children may be demonstrating signs of autism. However, the girl is less likely to be referred for testing. More research needs to be conducted in order to identify significant and reliable reasons why there is such a profound gender gap in autism.

Socioeconomic Status—Does it Matter?

The current research on the debate of whether children from lower or higher socioeconomic status (SES) are more likely to be diagnosed with autism appears to be variable. There is sufficient evidence on either side of the debate, ultimately raising questions such as: How does SES affect Autism diagnosis? Do children from lower SES backgrounds have higher rates of autism? Do families from higher SES backgrounds have higher rates of autism? What impact does SES have on early intervention, resources, and diagnosis?

The earliest studies of autism, by Kanner in 1943, concluded that the majority of families in his case study came from "intelligent families." Researchers have since attempted to prove that it is not intelligent families that have higher rates of autism. Rather they have better access to autism resources, resulting in more autism diagnoses. Many researchers attempted to utilize healthcare records but were often unable to gather enough information, resorting to school records instead. This finding raises the fact that individuals living in the United States do not have equal access to healthcare, which could lead to a sample bias in exploring SES differences (Rai et al., 2012). Interestingly, when researchers posed the same questions in other countries that have universal healthcare, the findings were very different. For example, in Denmark, after taking into account confounding variables such as risk factors, families with lower SES had higher rates of autism, but (Larsson et al., 2005; Rai et al., 2012) found the results not to be essential in the relationship between SES and autism. Rai and colleagues (2012) conducted a large matched-control study to further explore these questions using national health registers in Sweden while reducing case bias by looking at parental education, occupational class, and SES. They found that children from lower SES backgrounds and parents who worked manual labor jobs or did not get compensated by civil services had higher rates of autism. They did not find an association between the level of parental education and autism. It appears there are several potential risk factors or reasons why the United States demonstrated differing results compared to other countries. Possible causes could be due to higher SES families having better access to autism resources or to sampling bias in studying younger children, whereas lower SES children are often diagnosed later in life, thus limiting their ability to participate in national surveys (Fountain et al., 2012; Rai et al., 2012). There needs to be substantial research on the influence of SES and rates of autism.

Intersection of identities

A person with autism is considered to have a disability. Identities such as ethnicity or race, religion, sexual orientation, gender, nation of origin, and SES can place us in society for the rest of our lives. When we enter a room or begin speaking with friends, family, or even strangers, people make quick judgments based on our perceived, assumed, and expressed identities. The judgments we make are usually subconscious, but they can also be intentional and are often incorrect. Some of our identities may be of the majority, meaning in comparison to others, we are more similar to the people around us than different. Although it may not always be obvious, being part of a majority identity group places us in a seat of privilege. In short, privileges are social advantages that a person or specific group of people have been granted, such as protection or exemption against certain legal and social sanctions. In other words, someone with privilege has a right or advantage that another person or group does not have. The more majority identities we obtain, whether we were born into them or experience them over time, the more privilege we hold. Someone who holds a majority identity, such as a person who is racialized as white, can also fall into other minority population groups such as gender, religion, or SES. Take a moment to process how many of your identities are part of the majority or minority within your current social and geographic context. When a person has several majority identities, they have increased chances to navigate the world with less prejudice, discrimination, hate, and daily microaggressions. In contrast, a person who falls into one or many minority groups has a higher chance of experiencing mental health challenges due to living in a world that is not always accommodating or kind to people in minority groups. This phenomenon speaks to the reality of privilege. Although social climates are slowly changing for the better, people who hold minority identities still face daily stigma, discrimination, and prejudice. It is easier to enter the world by ignoring differences and leaning into our biases and subconscious beliefs. However, to ignore culture and privilege is to ignore the truths and the harm people in minority populations experience, further perpetuating the notion of invisibility. Not all people with autism consider themselves to have a "disability." However, once a person receives a diagnosis, they are placed into a category that comes with preconceived notions from the world. These preconceived beliefs can be harmful to individuals and families. Some people hold their disability status close to their identity, which can often be ignored due to the sometimes "invisible" appearance of autism. Sadly, some neurotypical people may say, "They don't look like they have autism." This microaggression can be extremely invalidating and add subconscious pressures for people to mask their autistic behaviors. For many people with autism, the diagnosis is a salient part of their identity. The point is, for some, the autism diagnosis can be fulfilling and positive. Ignoring its significance as a large part of someone can have damaging psychological effects.

Meyer (2003) examined this reality of minority stress. He created a model that speaks to the serious issues people of minority groups face and their impacts on psychological and physical well-being. Although the model was initially created to explore gender and sexual minority groups, Botha and Frost (2020) conducted a remarkable study utilizing the minority stress model to better understand how people on the spectrum experience their social identities having a disability and its connections to mental health. The researchers note the importance of understanding stigma and how it transforms to become harmful to the targeted group. Stigma is a process of labeling that places someone in a category based on perceived characteristics (Link & Phelan, 2013). Once a label is assigned, it is not the awareness of labels that becomes harmful but instead how society attaches meaning to that label, which further perpetuates its impact and long-term use (Botha & Frost, 2020; Link & Phelan, 2013). One study that interviewed students who did not have autism found that children shared several beliefs and stereotypes about people with autism. Nine out of ten stereotypes of autism were negative (Wood & Freeth, 2016). Having a diagnosis of autism, or being a person with a disability, can bring life-long social, educational, and political setbacks. These setbacks can be influenced, created, or even exaggerated by others having false beliefs about people with disabilities. Researchers hypothesize that being part of a minority group leads to more stressful life events while consequently having less access to appropriate resources to cope. Limited access to resources can be the result of social structures excluding minority groups. Social structures include state and government agencies that create programs and access to resources for more advantaged groups. After interviewing 111 participants about daily discrimination, victimization, internalized stigma, general life stressors, physically concealing autism traits, and overall well-being, Botha and Frost (2020) researchers found that individuals with autism, in fact, experience added minority stress, which thus affects their psychological well-being. More specifically, the stressors of having autism persisted beyond the effects of general minority stressors such as gender, sexual orientation, and religion. This means that the participants reported that having autism created more challenges for them than other cultural identities. This information is vital because it speaks to the clinical concerns the autism population needs from mental health professionals. The current research sheds light on the possible hidden impacts of minority stress that can overwhelmingly influence people on the spectrum. It may also be the case that families who obtain several minority identities experience similar negative impacts on their mental health and well-being. Additional research would need to be conducted to assess this claim. However, it is clear that a person with autism and a disability diagnosis is navigating the social world at a disadvantage intertwined with stigma and discrimination. It is the responsibility of clinicians, local and state agencies, families, and educators to support individuals with autism and their families through advocacy, allyship, psychoeducation, and equal access to resources.

When clinicians or mental health providers meet with families of autism, diversity factors and the intersections of identity must be considered and evaluated. Not every family will experience autism in the same way, especially if individuals are members of various minority groups. Consider working directly with a single parent who is Latinx, Roman Catholic, or a first-generation immigrant from a lower SES background. This parent may be experiencing several psychosocial stressors being part of several minority groups. A teacher or mental health provider must offer this parent appropriate support and understand that they might have fewer cognitive and financial resources. In other words, what might work or be helpful for one family, might not work for another when we consider various cultural factors that affect how families manage each day. The parent above might need additional resources, such as greater community support, patience, increased communication, and hands-on learning. This parent may not appear to be concerned about their child with autism because their current and more pertinent stressors involve providing for their family or experiencing racism in the workplace. What could appear at first glance as a parent who is uninvolved or incapable can look drastically different when we put on our diversity lens. It is essential when working with any family that one orient oneself to the diverse factors of that family, including their family makeup, mental health history, and who may live within the home. Different family types, such as an adoptive or a stepfamily, can provide us with information and insight into unique stressors that parents are juggling, all while attempting to support their child with autism. Since families exist within various systems, one must know how these systems are either supporting or burdening each member. In other words, one cannot effectively address autism if the surrounding environment is facing its own crisis.

How is Autism Treated?

Traditionally, autism has been viewed as an individual neurodevelopmental concern and is treated as such. An extensive literature review by Rogers and Vismara (2008) found through randomized controlled trials that one effective way to treat autism is through early interventions, specifically improving the severity of symptoms and overall developmental functioning. A version of early intervention is known as early intensive behavioral intervention (EIBI). This treatment modality is a form of behavioral therapy rooted in ABA, which is the most common treatment for autism. Some even believe ABA is the most effective intervention to treat autism (Matson et al., 2012). ABA is a combination of various psychosocial interventions that are rooted in behavioral theory to shape a person's behavior. The goal of ABA is to improve overall skills in communication, play, and daily living and reduce harmful behavior (Jensen & Sinclair, 2002). However, ABA lacks cultural awareness, diversity considerations, and the changing internal and external systems, including family and community support. Specifically, this book proposes a more effective, holistic, and systematic theory to treat autism and families. Although autism may only be diagnosed in one person, the entire family system is affected in unique ways. It is not uncommon that families and communities must work together to support a person on the spectrum, which includes extended family, schools, psychological services, and local agencies. Ecosystemic Structural Family Therapy (ESFT) is a systemic, strength-based family therapy model that has evolved from structural family therapy (Minuchin, 1974; Jones & Lindblad-Goldberg, 2008; Lindblad-Goldberg & Northey, 2013). Where ABA lacks particular components that are essential when working with autism, EFST is based on the belief that all behavior is a form of communication within a defined cultural context, that symptoms are due to the context of social interactions, and that families are always evolving as internal and external systems change over time. These are just a few key aspects of EFST. This model goes beyond the person with autism and treats the very structures that influence, maintain, and create change.

Conclusion

As autism research grows and advances, the way we think, understand, and treat autism should evolve with it. To better understand the spectrum itself and how diversity and culture influence individual experience, we have to be open-minded. One should be open to the possibility that as research evolves, we will have to challenge our previous beliefs about what we once knew. Autism is a neurodevelopmental disorder that can be observed on a spectrum of various social communication limitations, behavioral challenges, and restricted or repetitive patterns of behavior or interests and activities. Autism can impact a person and their family from the moment they obtain a formal diagnosis. It is clear that there is a disproportion of ethnoracial diagnoses of autism in people who identify as Latinx and other ethnic/racial groups. Institutions, schools, and medical practices should be well versed in the current research and literature about autism. If we ignore the gaps and limitations in research, we ignore very real issues within the assessment and treatment of autism. For example, the fact that there are limited numbers of bilingual-trained ABA therapists and culturally informed treatment models sheds light on shifts that need to be made within the field. We have to assume that there is always room for us to grow and become more informed. Treating autism through a cultural and inclusive lens requires meeting with the entire family system. Utilizing a systems approach promotes visibility for multiple identity factors that influence a person and their family's daily experiences. Teachers, researchers, and clinicians need to be informed about diversity impacts on the assessment and treatment of autism. Or, at the very least, be aware of personal biases and values that could influence how we perceive autism, what we know, and where our blind spots might be. For example, diversity factors greatly influence the diagnosis of autism, treatment options, and the availability of resources. Specifically, clinicians need to consider how treatment goals can intersect with cultural ideologies. The best way to understand cultural ideologies and beliefs is to meet with the entire family. Doing so also allows clinicians to observe relational, emotional, and structural dynamics unique to each family. This book will provide a rationale for the use of the ecosystemic structural family therapy model as the foundational treatment model. In addition, clear case examples and tailored interventions will be demonstrated for treating families on the autism spectrum.

References

American Psychiatric Association. (2013). Diagnostic and statistical manual of mental disorders (5th ed.).

Botha, M., & Frost, D. M. (2020). Extending the minority stress model to understand mental health problems experienced by the autistic population. *Society and Mental Health, 10*(1), 20–34.

Christensen, D. L. (2016). Prevalence and characteristics of autism spectrum disorder among children aged 8 years—autism and developmental disabilities monitoring network, 11 sites, United States, 2012. *MMWR. Surveillance Summaries, 65*.

Fountain, C., King, M. D., & Bearman, P. S. (2011). Age of diagnosis for autism: Individual and community factors across 10 birth cohorts. *Journal of Epidemiology & Community Health, 65*(6), 503–510.

Fountain, C., Winter, A. S., & Bearman, P. S. (2012). Six developmental trajectories characterize children with autism. *Pediatrics, 129*(5), e1112–e1120.

Geschwind, D. H. (2008). Advances in autism. *Annual Review of Medicine, 60*, 367. https://doi.org/10.1146/annurev.med.60.053107.121225

Grzadzinski, R., Huerta, M., & Lord, C. (2013). DSM-5 and autism spectrum disorders (ASDs): an opportunity for identifying ASD subtypes. *Molecular Autism, 4*, 1–6.

Hops, J., & Reschly, D. (2003). Referral rates for intervention or assessment. *Journal of Special Education, 37*, 67–80.

Jensen, V. K., & Sinclair, L. V. (2002). Treatment of autism in young children: Behavioral intervention and applied behavior analysis. *Infants & Young Children, 14*(4), 42–52.

Jones, C. W., & Lindblad-Goldberg, M. (2008). Ecosystemic structural family therapy: A primer. In K. Jordan (Ed.), *The quick theory reference guide: A resource for expert and novice mental health professionals* (pp. 331–347). Nova Science Publishers.

Kitzhaber, S. (2012). Interventions for multicultural children with autism. Retrieved from https://sophia.stkate.edu/msw_papers/118

Kanner, L. (1943). Autistic disturbances of affective contact. *Nervous Child, 2,* 217–250.

Lai, M., Lombardo, M. V., Auyeung, B., Chakrabarti, B., & Baron-Cohen, S. (2015). Sex/gender differences and autism: Setting the scene for future research. *Journal of the American Academy of Child & Adolescent Psychiatry, 54*(1), 11–24. https://doi.org/10.1016/j.jaac.2014.10.003

Larsson, H. J., Eaton, W. W., Madsen, K. M., Vestergaard, M., Olesen, A. V., Agerbo, E., ... & Mortensen, P. B. (2005). Risk factors for autism: Perinatal factors, parental psychiatric history, and socioeconomic status. *American Journal of Epidemiology, 161*(10), 916–925.

Lindblad-Goldberg, M., & Northey, W. F. (2013). Ecosystemic structural family therapy: Theoretical and clinical foundations. *Contemporary Family Therapy, 35,* 147–160.

Link, B. G., & Phelan, J. C. (2013). Labeling and stigma. In C. S. Aneshensel, J. C. Phelan, & A. Bierman (Eds.), *Handbook of the sociology of mental health* (2nd ed., pp. 525–541). Springer Science + Business Media. https://doi.org/10.1007/978-94-007-4276-5_25

Maenner, M. J., Warren, Z., Williams, A. R., et al. (2023). Prevalence and characteristics of autism spectrum disorder among children aged 8 years — Autism and developmental disabilities monitoring network, 11 Sites, United States, 2020. *MMWR Surveillance Summaries, 72*(No. SS-2), 1–14. http://dx.doi.org/10.15585/mmwr.ss7202a1

Maenner, M. J., Shaw, K. A., Baio, J., et al. (2020). Prevalence of autism spectrum disorder among children aged 8 years — Autism and developmental disabilities monitoring network, 11 Sites, United States, 2016. *MMWR Surveillance Summaries, 69*(No. SS-4), 1–12. http://dx.doi.org/10.15585/mmwr.ss6904a1

Matson, J. L., Turygin, N. C., Beighley, J., Rieske, R., Tureck, K., & Matson, M. L. (2012). Applied behavior analysis in autism spectrum disorders: Recent developments, strengths, and pitfalls. *Research in Autism Spectrum Disorders, 6*(1), 144–150.

Meyer, I. H. (2003). Prejudice, social stress, and mental health in lesbian, gay, and bisexual populations: Conceptual issues and research evidence. *Psychological Bulletin, 129*(5), 674.

Minuchin, S. (1974). Families and family therapy. Cambridge, MA: Harvard University.

Morrier, M. J., Hess, K. L., & Heflin, L. J. (2008). Ethnic disproportionality in students with autism spectrum disorders. *Multicultural Education, 16*(1), 31–38.

National Research Council. (2001). Educating children with autism. Committee on educational interventions for children with autism. In C. Lord & J. P. McGee, eds. *Division of Behavioral and Social Sciences and Education.* Washington, DC: National Academy Press

Rai, D., Lewis, G., Lundberg, M., Araya, R., Svensson, A., Dalman, C., ... & Magnusson, C. (2012). Parental socioeconomic status and risk of offspring autism spectrum disorders in a Swedish population-based study. *Journal of the American Academy of Child & Adolescent Psychiatry, 51*(5), 467–476.

Rogers, S. J., & Vismara, L. A. (2008). Evidence-based comprehensive treatments for early autism. *Journal of Clinical Child & Adolescent Psychology, 37*(1), 8–38.

Sen, E., & Yurtsever, S. (2007). Difficulties experienced by families with disabled children. *Journal for Specialists in Pediatric Nursing, 12*(4), 238–252.

Wang, Y., Kang, S., Ramirez, J., & Tarbox, J. (2019). Multilingual diversity in the field of applied behavior analysis and autism: A brief review and discussion of future directions. *Behavior Analysis in Practice, 12*(4), 795–804. https://doi.org/10.1007/s40617-019-00382-1

Wood, C., & Freeth, M. (2016). Students' stereotypes of autism. *Journal of Educational Issues, 2*(2), 131–140.

2 Ecological Systems Approach
Ecosystemic Structural Family Therapy

Scott Browning

Families on the Autism Spectrum (FotAS)

While there is a huge variation in symptoms and concerns across the variety of families in which at least one member is on the autism spectrum, there are similarities. The severity of symptoms ranges widely, but it is common a family will deal with an individual who has rigid behavior, some repetition or compulsion, and a lack of social skills, who demonstrates language issues, and who shows volatility. Therefore, just as it would be inaccurate to expect that any one treatment is appropriate for all individuals on the autism spectrum, it would also follow that family therapy will vary as well. However, the needs of these families share enough similarities that for the purpose of describing therapy to assist these families, this book continues to use the term, Families on the Autism Spectrum (FotAS).

This chapter is intended as a guide to engage and treat such families. Greenspan and Wieder (1998) clearly state that if a family is fully engaged in the life of the member on the spectrum, benefits to the family are likely. In other words, this book supports the idea that addressing concerns experienced by these families is particularly useful due to the frequent possible miscommunications and differences of opinion that exist. Someone on the autism spectrum has a unique trajectory of development: it is part of this diagnosis. Therefore, traditional parenting manuals are not particularly useful to the autism spectrum disorder family population.

General Factors for the Family on the Autism Spectrum

Developmentally predictable stages or milestones are relevant to FotAS due to their absence. For many parents, referring to experts who outline the developmental stages of the growing child is a standard rite of passage. But, for the parent of a child on the spectrum, these charts are not only inaccurate, but they are also a painful reminder of the way in which a

DOI: 10.4324/9781003451266-2

developmental disorder, in this case autism, impacts the child at various points along the lifespan.

FotAS, by definition, create their own sociopolitical context. Most FotAS need to engage in some activism, even if it is just doing the occasional Autism Walk. But, most FotAS are able to channel some energy into building an autism-friendly community. The environment in Western culture has become more open and tolerant of special needs. However, even in a more compassionate world, an "autism-friendly" or "disability-friendly" community is difficult to achieve. Most people existing in the neurotypical world have little one-on-one involvement with someone on the spectrum; thus, they have limited, academic understanding of autism. Altiere and von Kluge (2009) conducted a qualitative study exploring the struggles and successes of families on the spectrum. They found that the family on the spectrum, generally, will feel systemic pressure to isolate (Altiere & von Kluge, 2009). To counter this inclination, FotAS need to find environments in which one's child's unusual behavior is totally accepted.

A sense of community is desirable for all people, but the family on the autism spectrum often is challenged in establishing a sense of community (Gutstein, 2000). If one feels unaccepted, the tendency is to isolate. For many FotAS, the temptation to isolate is born out of feeling unwelcome at community events, restaurants, typical sporting events, religious services, and extended family gatherings. While family therapy is designed to assist the family in addressing the concerns they are experiencing, at times, typical responses, such as increased isolation, may be addressed as a common concern.

Family Therapy

The family therapist should be aware that for many FotAS, treatment options are being brought up by friends, family, schools, aides, and professionals. While this may sound supportive, and usually the information is meant to be helpful, the result is that often these families feel bombarded with all the things that they could be doing, with editorial comments consisting of a sense that if they did "this one," things would get better. Thus, the family therapist, while certainly aware of the variety of treatments available for individuals with autism, will be careful not to be one more voice in the chorus of ideas, but rather to serve as a manager who assists the family in critiquing what might be worth trying, what might be ignored, and how to deal with the well-meaning people creating a cacophony of suggestions.

Due to the particular combination of miscommunication, anxiety, and volatility for those on the autism spectrum, the appearance of a crisis needs to be normalized to these families. Certainly, one can never become complacent about a crisis, but shifting one's reaction to these predictable crises can be helpful. For example, a child with autism could get lost in a crowded place. Certainly, modern technology helps keep track of us all, but at the fair, a phone might be in mom's purse due to the upside-down nature of the ride and the child could wander the wrong way from the exit. A typical reaction of blaming the other parent or the neurotypical sibling is not helpful. Families on the autism spectrum may have to shift their reactions from blame to problem-solving and communication. In the end, screaming at someone who was supposed to follow a child every step of the way ignores the unique challenges of being a FotAS. Blame takes families one step further from solutions as a team.

This short list of common occurrences for the FotAS is intended to assist the family therapist in normalizing or accepting many of the events and dilemmas that occur for these families. Normalizing is a term used to describe people going through some process (e.g., grief, remarriage, depression, etc.) that certain symptoms and challenges are typical. Thus, normalizing or acceptance does not suggest that the concern raised is not problematic, just that it is common. For many people, just knowing others experience the same concerns makes the situation less scary. Normalizing should not be overused, but helping people see how "normal" a reaction is, can assist an FotAS in reaching acceptance with less judgment and shame. Certainly, there are aspects that deserve emotional upset, blaming, and confusion. However, when some of these events lose their emotional force, the family feels less out of control. For example, knowing that one's child will need to exit the restaurant the second the food on their plate is finished, allows the parents the latitude to decide how they will still enjoy a night out, although the rules are now idiosyncratic.

Why Ecosystemic Structural Family Therapy Fits the Needs of the Family on the Autism Spectrum

Ecosystemic Structural Family Therapy (ESFT) is a widely utilized, strongly validated treatment approach to families. The model is an elegant revision of the Structural Family Therapy Model (Minuchin, 1974). ESFT utilizes the attention the therapist pays to hierarchy, coalitions, and boundaries from Structural Family Therapy and adds significant attention to the creation of emotional regulation and the strengthening of attachment. ESFT has been established as an Evidence Supported Practice through multiple trials with real-life families (Jones & Lindblad-Goldberg, 2002; Jones, 2019). The approach uses two styles to deliver treatment. For highly dysfunctional families that need to be treated in a home-based approach, the model incorporates a team of two therapists in order to fully align with the various members and the different clinical issues at hand for those families. However, the model is also well designed for what might be considered less dysfunctional families, within which the FotAS generally falls. In these cases, the typical treatment is a single therapist (under supervision) working at an office or online with the family.

The therapist, working in this modality, begins with overarching questions, originally from Structural Family Therapy, that need to be understood to focus the treatment. The first question is: Is there a central authority in the family? Second, if there is a central authority, is it a single person or a co-parental team? The third question is: Are the boundaries between the generations established and stable?

In addition to these foundational questions, the therapist (in following an ecosystemic approach), is addressing attachment and emotional regulation. Attachment has become a widely used term in modern therapy approaches. While the term has a historical meaning determined by the research of Bowlby (1998), it has come to be a shorthand for representing a positive, trusting relationship. While it is a luxury to have good attachment throughout a family, at minimum, people need at least one person in their lives that they know is trustworthy, caring, and supportive. Thus, the therapist is looking to determine if that is true for the members of the family in front of them. Family therapy has as a general goal, the mission of reattaching people who no longer feel, or never experienced, a positive attachment.

It is important to discuss some basics of family treatment that have evolved over the history of systems therapy. While the notion of seeing all family members together still remains one of the methods of family treatment, the use of subsystems (seeing the family in smaller groupings) has increased dramatically over the last fifteen years (Browning & van Eeden-Moorefield, 2022). The subsystem approach is particularly helpful when seeing warring family members simply increases the perception of being stuck and untrusting. Family therapy relies on enough goodwill that people are capable of listening to one another. Working with subsystems allows the therapist to hear the concerns of each person, join with all people, and assist these family members in calming down enough to consider alternatives that might improve the entire situation for the family.

Treatment: Step by Step

Treatment with the family begins with an initial meeting. Historically, the rule of thumb had been to bring in as many family members as possible. That rule has shifted and family therapy now takes the position that one should start with those family members who are an important subsystem for an understanding of the problem and systemic functioning. Thus, it might just be the parents in the first session, the parents and one child, or any combination of family members. Due to traditional consent protocol, clinicians worry about clients' hearing secrets that might affect clinical progress, so they fear subsystem meetings. However, this is easily dealt with by having family members sign consent (or in the case of minors, assent) that allows the therapist to determine whether some secrets are damaging if left unknown. Then, over time, a method is determined for sharing information that is unhealthy for the family as a whole. Doing systems therapy, one sees the whole family as the client. Of course, traditional legal sharing of information in the case of abuse or suicide, remains ever present.

In the initial meeting, the therapist will begin to draw a genogram with the participation of those there. The genogram will serve as a tool in assisting in forming a case conceptualization. While creating the genogram, the therapist asks about the concerns, as well as the strengths, of the family. While no family therapy model is considered the only approach, this book highlights the ESFT approach as particularly useful. Thus, in keeping with the foundational questions raised earlier, the therapist will assess the alliance between caregivers. Often, the parents are the caregivers, but certainly, other compositions are common. If there is a single caregiver (e.g., parent or grandparent), with no other person involved, the focus shifts to gaining some support either from within the extended family or from professional assistance. In the situation of two or more people involved in the caregiving of children (at least one on the autism spectrum for this example), the quality of the alliance is closely examined. Do the caregivers respect each other's opinions? Or, is the alliance fractured due to a perception that the caregivers are not in agreement on parenting style?

The therapist's goal will shift in response to the perceived alliance of the caregivers. If the caregivers are not in agreement regarding parenting, it will be necessary to remain neutral and learn about each person's philosophy of parenting a child on the autism spectrum. Is the difference due to distinctly different relationships with the child, or is the difference based on a fundamental disagreement on what parenting approach is both effective and helpful to the child's growth? This disagreement must be handled carefully. The therapist needs to avoid alienating either caregiver early in the relationship. A discussion, with examples, will help the therapist gain an understanding of each person's parenting philosophy and comfort with the issues present in this child's behavioral presentation. This chapter specifically examines parenting with the child on the autism spectrum. While parenting issues may be problematic in those cases in which there is another sibling, who is not on the spectrum, traditional family therapy texts have covered that topic thoroughly (Nichols & Schwartz, 2018).

Sessions with each caregiver separately will often assist the therapist to support those components of the caregiver's methods that are effective, while also challenging those caregiving procedures that are judged to be unhelpful. These meetings with individuals have the goal of both gaining alliance with the parent, and finding a rationale to support particular interventions.

As with all co-parents, it is hoped that some positive relationship between these caregivers exists outside of parenting. That relationship may be as a loving couple, or a healthy mother-daughter bond that is not entirely dictated by the parenting issues. For example, looking at the genogram for Ryan's family (see Figure 2.1), it is clear that Ryan's parents are in conflict with each other, on occasion, but generally are close with Ryan. Ryan's discomfort with wet hair, leading him to refuse to shower, is a significant point of conflict.

Figure 1, Genogram of Ryan's Family

Clinical Case: Ryan's Family

Therapist: Let's start where you both agree, you both want Ryan not to smell, at home or at school. (Determine some mutual goal.)

Mother: Yeah, that is true.

Father: I agree, but a full shower does more than just wash off the stink.

Mother: You're are not the one usually wrestling with him into the shower.

Father: That's true, but I have done it and at the end, he is clean.

Therapist: Is it fair to say that there is no winner in this situation. Ryan is either going to fight against a wet head or be dirty?

Mother: Well, not exactly, sometimes a sponge bath will keep him from smelling.

Father: He still needs to shampoo sometimes.

Mother: I know!

Therapist: Is there any system that would reduce your conflict with each other and largely accomplish your goal?

While the discussion continues, Beth and Bill (Ryan's parents) begin to work as a team rather than simply complaining about the other. Sometimes recognizing a place where the family is stuck and accepting that a perfect solution does not exist, enables the automatic rejection of the other co-parent to lessen.

In the example just discussed, the therapist is doing the following steps: supporting that there can be a mutual goal, accepting the co-parents as both invested and worthwhile, reducing the emotional reactivity

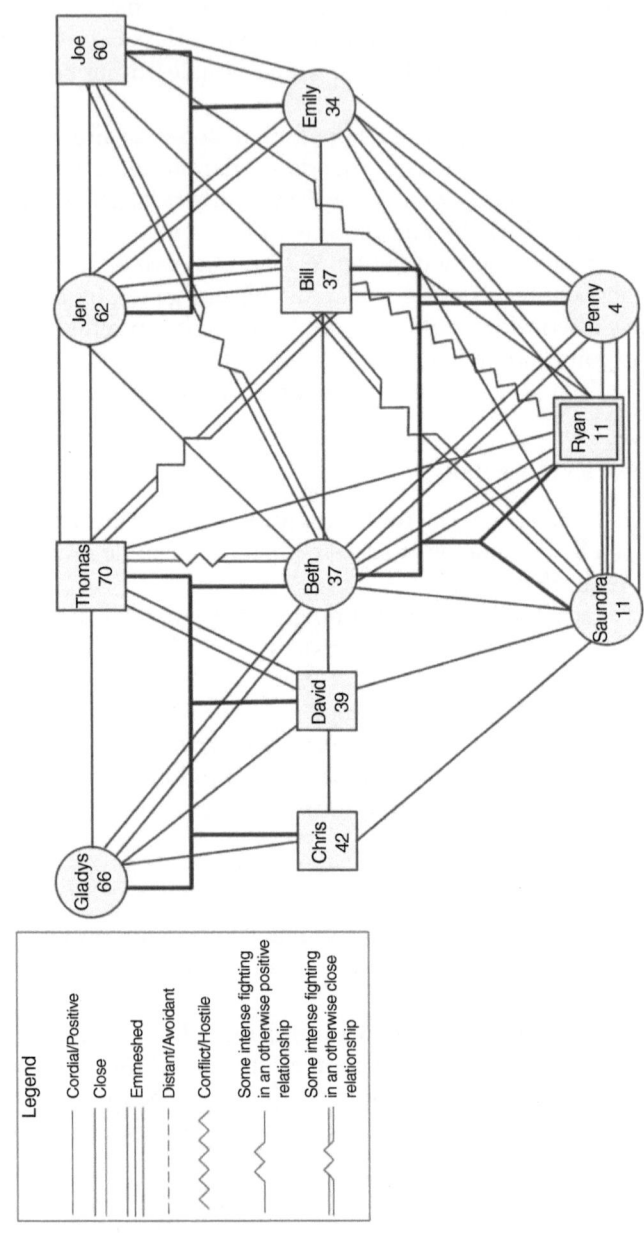

Figure 2.1 Ryan's family.

between the co-parents, and examining possible behavioral changes across the system.

Systems therapy works on a variety of goals with the interventions provided. A critical goal in ESFT is to increase the caregiver's emotional availability to their children. In essence, emotional availability will increase with improvement of a bond. The child on the autism spectrum can challenge a caregiver in feeling close. Many traditional adult mechanisms to increase connection to a child are ineffective with a child on the autism spectrum. For example, the common practice of the father's roughhousing or tickling a neurotypical child to "break the ice," will often fail spectacularly with the child with autism. Being in "one's own world" makes the sudden increase of sensation shocking and unpleasant to the highly sensitive child, whereas the neurotypical child often loves the increase in safe intensity.

Continuing with the case of Ryan (see Figure 2.1), there is conflict indicated between Bill (the dad) and Ryan. It is safe to speculate that the symbol representing conflict can also be interpreted as indicating a lack of emotional availability. Improving this relationship is of critical importance to the success of the case, overall. As seen from the previous therapy example, Ryan's sensitivity to a wet head is one area of conflict; however, just as problematic between Dad and Ryan is the lack of any positive bond. While Bill claims to love Ryan, and there is no reason to suggest this in not true, Bill acknowledges that he is chronically disappointed in having no bonding activity (e.g., tossing a ball, sports, going out together), thus leading Bill to feel angry and a failure as a dad.

Clinically, the goal in this situation would be to assist Bill and Ryan to build a relationship based on more than fighting over showering. It is in this work that one utilizes treatment ideas advocated by experts in autism. For this example, the work of Stanley Greenspan is utilized.

Greenspan's Floortime was a unique shift away from strict behaviorism and toward more interactional treatment (Greenspan & Wieder, 1998). In this case, Floortime is taught to Bill to assist him in gaining competence in learning how to relate to his son on the autism spectrum.

Floortime advocates that the individual on the autism spectrum is in a position of power. Whatever this individual does, no matter how seemingly random or disconnected the actions are, the adult follows the child's lead. The child pushing a stick across the floor is seen as creating an activity. They are actively pushing the stick, and the parent, Bill, in this example, can begin to comment ("Wow, that stick is going from one wall to the other") or play with Ryan. Unlike typical play, in Floortime the adult does anything to become part of the action. One might put their hand on the floor so the stick has to go over it, or one might grab another stick and follow.

Bill is taught to avoid coaching Ryan on the right way to push a stick, or a way that the game is more interesting to Bill. Rather, the entire goal of Floortime is to have Bill, on the floor, learning to be with Ryan and see his actions as something of interest. Often, after doing this activity over a number of days, even highly disconnected children (which Ryan is not) begin to acknowledge Dad's presence and may even look to be enjoying the interaction.

Therapy with Bill includes hearing his frustration, showing empathy for the loss of the son he may have hoped for, and encouraging him that a relationship, although not the one envisioned, is possible and can be enjoyable. The following example demonstrates this process.

Therapist: Do you wish to learn a way to gain a bond with Ryan?

Bill: Well, of course, I don't like feeling that Ryan is a stranger to me.

Therapist: There is a process called Floortime that can be very effective in building relationships. Would you be willing to try?

Bill: Yes, I am willing to try, but it is not like I have not tried to get to know Ryan.

Therapist: I know, I am not suggesting that. What I am saying is that building these relationships with people on the autism spectrum is not obvious and does not follow many of the rules we grew up with.

Bill: Like I said, yes.

Therapist: Great. We are going to use a method called Floortime, invented by Stanley Greenspan. In essence, Ryan is in charge of your activities. Whatever he does, you show interest, try a running commentary, and try to insert yourself whenever you can. We will start together. Follow my lead, and I will begin to move out when you are getting it.

Clinical Case: Max's Family

In keeping with systemic therapy, treating the FotAS follows a standard family therapy truism: expanding the treatment to include extended family when possible. One of the four systemic common factors (interventions common across all systems models) (Sprenkle, Davis & Lebow, 2009) is the belief that being open to expanding treatment to include more family members is consistently helpful. This can be particularly important in FotAS since the member on the autism spectrum is frequently a bit of a mystery to extended family members. While exceptions occur, especially as autism becomes more common and accepted, the confusion surrounding autism can have the effect of pulling families apart or at least decreasing family get-togethers. It is not uncommon to hear grandparents express a desire to be close to a grandchild on the autism spectrum but feel unsure how to achieve this since efforts at connecting with these children can be challenging. While it may appear that grandparents are not working at joining with their grandchild, it must be understood that the child may also be uncertain how to make a connection as well. Parents may also be a factor in that they have achieved a level of competence at relating to their child on the autism spectrum, but are frustrated with the attitudes and behaviors of adult siblings and their parents, thus leading to an unstated message that "only I know how to relate to Tommy."

Addressing the extended family clinically in these families is usually a relatively safe and effective intervention. ESFT is perpetually working to promote growth in the family. In keeping with the ESFT goals, the incorporation of extended family organizes the family and increases emotional connection. Given that older generations are frequently confused by the behaviors and comments of their grandchildren on the autism spectrum, assisting these families to be connected to extended family members clearly is in the service of building solid relationships. While including extended family members increases the likelihood that the child on the spectrum is more central to the whole family, this intervention usually, at minimum, helps extended family members understand the situation of the child's parents.

Max's family is an important exploration of working with the extended family. As shown in Figure 2.2, no hostility or conflict is represented in the genogram toward Max. At first glance, this would suggest generally cordial relations. However, in the situation of a non-speaking family member, cordial may simply mean that the extended family smiles and tries to be nice toward and about Max. It does not necessarily represent a relationship in the manner that "cordial" is usually used. Admittedly, relating to non-speaking people is challenging, and many people are intimidated about even beginning to imagine a relationship without language. The one exception to this cordial pattern is Charles, one grandfather who is distant from Max and openly shows some hostility to his presence in the home when Max and his parents are visiting.

The intervention utilized here is driven more by a desire of Sally, Max's mother, to be able to be comfortable in visiting her family and her in-laws while in the company of Max. As Sally stated, "I don't need my family to know Max the way I do, but I need them to understand him enough that they recognize that Phillip (Max's father) and I need to pave the way to avoid upset and turmoil." In other words, while Sally would love to teach her sister to be able to sit with Max and have some relationship with him, she would be satisfied with knowing that Janet (Sally's sister) is a teammate in managing Max in stressful situations. Therefore, family therapy was utilized to create a deeper understanding of Max with a select

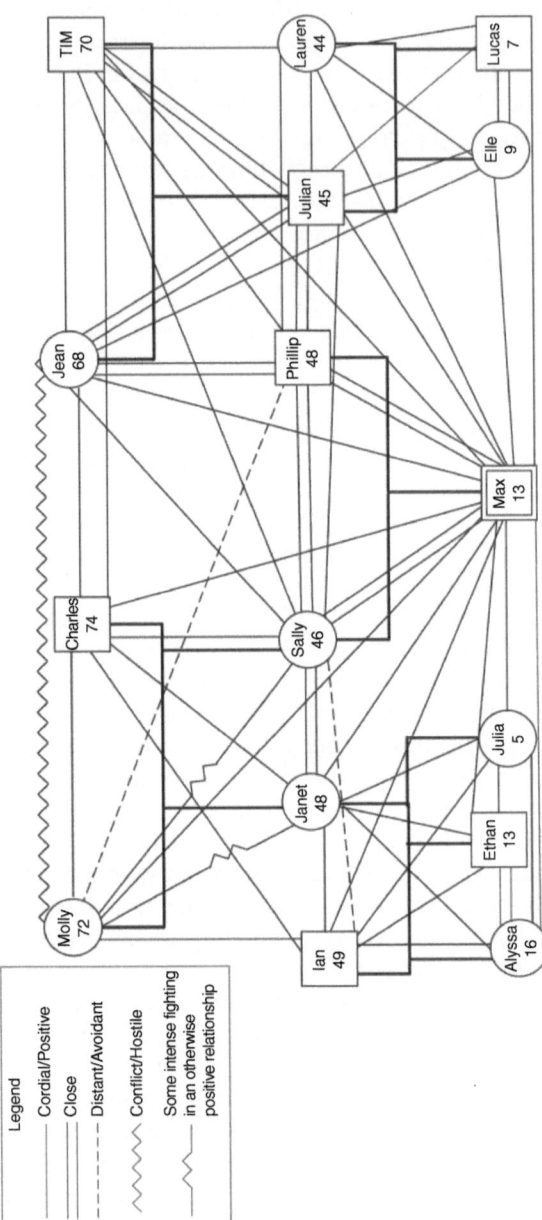

Figure 2.2 Max's family.

few family members. This process had the positive effect of calming Max since he perceived a few more people seemed to understand his needs, and clearly comforted Sally and Phillip.

Sally was asked in therapy to identify the one or two family members that she wanted to join, what she called "The Max Team." Janet was the primary choice for Sally since Janet had even said she wanted to be more involved and helpful. The beginning of this part of treatment involved meeting with Sally and Phillip to determine exactly what Janet should know about Max, and any hints of ways in which one can "be with" Max in a natural manner. In a sense, a parent of a child on the autism spectrum can create a "user's manual" of their child. What does this child enjoy? What to do if this child is upset? How to understand their basic needs? How does the parent describe the "full person inside" the outer presentation of the child? In this case, the therapist showed respect for the fact that Sally and Phillip were Max experts. This expertise could be shared with people interested in joining this team. Once the team has expanded, even by a single additional person, family visits are less desperate and overwhelming.

Once the parent meeting had determined what could be shared to assist Janet, the meeting with Janet was scheduled. The agenda for the meeting was made clear by Sally telling Janet exactly what the session was aiming to achieve, and Janet agreed. Choosing one member of a family is not rejecting the others. Certainly, anyone wishing to be on "Team Max" was welcome, but often, such interventions need to begin with one individual. The problem with attempting to do such a meeting with a wider family audience is that other topics often intrude. People wishing to apologize for not showing more interest, for miscommunication about Max and family get-togethers and such topics, often push their way into larger meetings and dilute the initial goal.

Thus, the following example reflects the content of the meeting with the therapist, Sally, Phillip, and Sally's sister, Janet.

Therapist: Janet, so nice to meet you, thanks for agreeing to be part of Team Max.

Janet: (chuckling) Yeah, this is a team that I want to join. But I am curious about what it will actually involve.

Therapist: What has Sally told you?

Janet: She says that it is hard to visit my folks since people don't understand why Max seems so removed in some ways, and so powerful in others.

Sally: Yeah, people are fine about Max until we have to jump up and avert a tantrum, then they are annoyed and think that Phillip and I are spoiling him and not holding him responsible. It is crazy.

Therapist: Sally, can you, or you, Phillip, if you prefer, explain why you are on eggshells with Max sometimes?

Sally: Sure, that is easy. He is a kid that if his mood shifts, or he starts to feel anxious, he will lose it. He may not speak, but he can scream, and he can throw things.

Janet: I am curious about that. Does he know what he is doing when he does that?

Therapist: This is exactly why these meetings are important. Sometimes these issues can't get discussed calmly in the middle of a meltdown. Sally, Phillip, any answer for Janet?

Phillip: It may be the wrong question. We are not sure if he is totally aware, but we know what calms him, know when he is happy, and keeping him calm and happy is our goal, even if it seems like we are spoiling him. He is not comfortable in social settings, except maybe at Special Olympics, when people seem happy to engage him. I think he feels overwhelmed at your parents' house. People yell at him like he is deaf; they never seem to know how to just accept him.

Sally: It is not better at your relatives.

Phillip: I know, I am not comparing, I am just frustrated. I am not mad at you, Janet, I swear.

Janet: No, I get it. It is just so confusing. Mom wants to be a good grandmother, I want to be a good aunt, but we have no idea how to actually do that.

Sally: I noticed you did not say that Dad wants to be a good grandfather.

Janet: He does not know what he thinks about Max.

Therapist: That is why Janet is here alone. The topic of a special needs child or grandchild generates strong feelings. Let's stay with helping Janet understand Max, and what can help you all make these occasional visits easier and happier. When you need to jump up to attend to Max, what would be helpful for Janet to do?

Sally: (Looking at Janet) Yeah, if you could say that Max will calm down and that it is nothing they did, and it would make us happy if people realize that we need (and want) to help him stay happy and calm.

Janet: Can you explain this ahead of time to Dad?

Therapist: Can you help me understand the issue around being straight with your father?

Janet: He keeps trying to guess what Sally and Phillip did to have Max be as he is. And, if I try to get people just to chill, it seems to make him angry, like we are giving up. But he does not really want much to do with Max.

Therapist: (Looking between Sally and Phillip) Would your parents (on both sides) be willing to be invited to a session?

Sally: I think my mom and Phillip's mom would come, maybe his dad.

Phillip: They would both come in. But I am not sure how this would go.

At this point, therapy moves into a consultation period. The therapist becomes entirely collaborative regarding the next appointments. In subsystem-based therapy (Browning & van Eeden-Moorefield, 2022), the selection of those invited is planned. The question the therapist asks themselves is, "What subsystem would provide a useful step in this family's healing?" In the case of Max and his family, the choice was exactly what Sally and Phillip agreed would be useful, a parent meeting. If Phillip's father does not show, that is his right. No one is forced into treatment. In making this decision, the next critical step is to create the agenda, and have all involved agreeing with the plan. It is here that the therapist's expertise is used. The therapist suggests some specific goals for this meeting. The goals are then edited by Sally and Phillip (and often new goals are added).

The session then shifts to determining safety. In the following section, the safety of this meeting is discussed.

Therapist: What do I need to know about the places this kind of meeting might go overboard? In other words, are there significant triggers that make people react emotionally?

Phillip: Whether Charles (Sally's father) comes or not, his view that we did something wrong, and we are still doing something wrong, pervades the whole family. He actually said it out loud in front of both families.

Sally: He is an ass when he is drunk. And he believes what he says.

Therapist: Okay, Charles' needs will be examined at some point. Maybe we can soften him. But for now, let's plan for the actual meeting. If all three come, do your in-laws get along, basically?

Sally: Yeah, they like my dad too, actually.

Therapist: Okay, let's talk through the agenda with safety in mind.

Phillip: What do you mean, safety?

Therapist: How do we not hurt anyone? We want to educate and conduct therapy, but we need to make sure no one is hurt. For example, if Charles does not come, we need to make sure your mother (looking at Sally), does not feel attacked about Charles not being there. This needs to be about understanding Max, recognizing the hurt and loss, as a family, and making the best of being a family with a non-speaking member.

Therapist: What I would like to do is give a brief lecture on autism and a clear path toward becoming a member of Team Max. This makes it clear that even just by helping you two (looking at Sally and Phillip), someone becomes a member of Team Max. I would then like to go over some examples of things that work, and why they work. Then I would move toward therapy. Having you all do a lot more talking.

Over the next few weeks, the parents were invited. To the surprise of Sally and Phillip, Charles did agree to come. As mentioned, the therapist starts as an educator. Emotions can wait in this family. So much of this family's life is stressful; therapy should be focused, helpful, and positive. If the family had a mission statement, it would go something like this, "Being a member of Team Max means that I take an interest in what Max is doing; I support people who love Max, and possibly interact with Max." The therapist is making the point that the family needs to communicate, care about each other, and yet accept that having Max in the family is still a significant burden, at times.

The following section is the initial meeting with Sally, Phillip, and all four parents.

Therapist: It's so nice to meet you all. I am Dr. Scott Browning, and I appreciate you all being here. The primary goal today is to gain a greater understanding of how Max goes through life. Also, we want to help people support each other, knowing the many challenges (and gifts) that having Max in your life brings.

Charles: I resent the idea that there are any gifts to having Max.

Phillip: See, he can't go two minutes without...

Therapist: Okay, let's get started. Max was born normally and no signs of autism appeared until he was age two. He made noises that sounded close to words, but never really spoke. He can communicate with the Picture Exchange Communication System [PECS] but he does not do it often. His comprehension is good. He can understand much of what you say, but that is hard to assess. He has a wide range of emotions. He can be happy, sad, angry, bored, and excited. Sometimes he tantrums. Usually, the reason for the tantrum is clear, a loud noise, a surprise, but sometimes the reason for the tantrum is never determined. Non-speaking is the term used for individuals like Max, rather than nonverbal. Like any parent, Sally and Phillip measure life satisfaction with Max doing okay and having a nice life. It is just that this mission is different from most parent/child relationships.

Therapist: Phillip, can you explain your perspective, and do so without comment about others, just what works for you to have a real relationship with Max?

As one reads that excerpt, the issue that Charles brought up feels heavy and hanging in the room.

It will be necessary to return to that, but the therapist needs to assess whether the four parents (to varying degrees) seem interested in becoming part of Team Max. The issue of Charles' comment is perfect for a daughter-father subsystem session. While Phillip will certainly be part of this conversation, it is best to have conversations like this between two people from a distance.

Therapist: Charles and Sally, thank you for coming in together. Given the tensions that have emerged since Max's diagnosis, is there anything you two still talk about that is a shared interest?

Charles: We still go bird-watching once a year. Down the shore.

Sally: Dad, I agree, and that is fun. It is just your feelings about Max; when he is around you, it is really hard on me, Phillip, and Max.

Charles: I am not sure Max notices.

Therapist: Sally, can you explain to your dad how you read Max's moods?

Sally: I mean, Dad, it is like telepathy. I see in his eyes that he is starting to freak out. I know it is disruptive, but jeez...

Therapist: Thanks, Sally, that is interesting. So, can you really read what Max is thinking at some level?

Sally: Yeah, at some level. I don't know what exactly he is thinking, but I can tell calm and happy from about to blow up.

Therapist: Is that something you could teach your parents?

Sally: I guess. Here is the problem: having them try in the beginning will make it worse. It is not their fault, Max is going to blow up more with more people interacting with him. But it is worth it since the blowups will fade once he knows you get him, again, to some level.

Therapist: Charles, if you knew that starting a real relationship with Max would be hard at first but would ultimately result in Sally feeling better and even you feeling better, would that be worth it to you?

Charles: I guess I have some concerns that the tantrums that come when I try to connect with Max will not really improve since I don't see him that often. But I don't want Sally or Phillip to think that we don't realize how hard it is to raise Max.

Sally: I think you mean that in a nice way, Dad, but sometimes Phillip and I don't want to be just pitied. Sometimes we just want people in the trenches with us.

Therapist: Team Max?

Sally: Yeah, exactly.

Charles: What if your mother and I could try this together and we find a way to see him more often?

Sally: I would be really grateful. I can't guarantee anything, but I know that Phillip and I can read Max, can comfort Max, and we can enjoy Max. I know that we will always be the team captains, but to have some support (which is starting with Janet) would be so great.

Treatment proceeded with engaging both Charles and Molly, Max's grandmother. The system was stabilized by helping Charles and Molly be good grandparents. Good family therapy makes people more stable. People understand the basic systems theory; they know their family affects multiple aspects of their lives. Janet, Max's aunt, is needed to support Charles and Molly, her parents. Having Janet on Team Max means that she can coach or just hang out while Charles and Molly are asked to communicate with Max.

Family therapy can go in multiple directions. While the therapist is helping people to be clear about their opinions and listen to others, it is the creation of a familial bond that is the ultimate goal. In using the evidence-supported approach, Ecosystemic Structural Family Therapy, a clinician can be assured that they are conducting treatment that is likely to be beneficial to the family on the autism spectrum.

References

Altiere, M. J., & Kluge, S. (2009). Searching for acceptance: Challenges encountered raising a child with autism. *Journal of Intellectual & Developmental Disability*, 34(2), 142–152. Doi:10.1080/13668250902845202

Bowlby, J. (1998). The nature of the child's tie to his mother. *International Journal of Psychoanalysis*, 39, 350–373.

Browning, S., & van Eeden-Moorefield, B. (2022). *Treating the Contemporary Family*. Washington, DC: American Psychological Association.

Greenspan, S., & Wieder, S. (1998). *The Child with Special Needs: Encouraging Intellectual and Emotional Growth*. Reading, MA: A Merloyd Lawrence Book.

Gutstein, S. E. (2000). *Autism Aspergers: Solving the Relationship Puzzle*. Arlington, TX: Future Horizons.

Jones, C. W. (2019). *Setting the Stage for Change: An Ecosystemic Approach to In-Home Family Based Treatment* (2nd Edition)Bala Cynwyd, PA: The Center for Family Based Training.

Jones, C. W., & Lindblad-Goldberg, M. (2002). Ecosystemic family therapy. In F. Kaslow (Series Ed.), & R. Massey and S. Massey (Volume Eds.). *Comprehensive Handbook of Psychotherapy: Vol. III, Interpersonal, Humanistic, and Existential Models*. New York, NY: John Wiley & Sons.

Minuchin, S. (1974). *Families & Family Therapy*. Cambridge, MA: Harvard University Press.

Nichols, M. P., & Schwartz, R. C. (2018). *Family Therapy: Concepts and Methods* (7th ed.). Needham Heights, MA: Allyn & Bacon.

Sprenkle, D. H., Davis, S., & Lebow, J. L. (2009). *Common Factors in Couple and Family Therapy*. New York, NY: Guilford Press.

3 The Autism Trait Scale (ATS)
A Clinical Instrument

Scott Browning

The Autism Trait Scale (ATS) was created in 2009 as a tool intended to clarify the presentation of autism spectrum disorder (ASD). For years, the common language of autism has been to describe those on the autism spectrum as either low functioning, medium functioning, or high functioning. Before that, the diagnostic category of Asperger's syndrome specified a person on the autism spectrum but usually suggested[1] a highly intelligent person for whom some of the classic autistic behaviors were present. However, this diagnostic category was flawed, and in 2013, the *Diagnostic Statistical Manual* (5th Edition) (American Psychiatric Association, 2013) removed the term "Asperger's" as a diagnostic category. At that point, the tri-part system was introduced and has remained stable. While more specific as to the characteristics, in essence, Level 1 is high functioning, Level 2 is moderate functioning, and Level 3 is low functioning. While this classification is helpful for researchers needing to establish basic categories, the average person is still provided with minimal context upon hearing that someone on the autism spectrum is high, medium, or low functioning.

The ATS is designed to fill in this gap. The scale allows a therapist or assessor to create a profile that highlights a comprehensive evaluation of strengths and challenges. The use of a graph with data points provides a profile that greatly increases one's understanding of the nature of the individual on the spectrum. As this chapter will highlight, using this tool is not intended as a method to determine the diagnosis of ASD; rather, this tool is used with family members, teachers, aides, and therapists to give a fuller description of the individual to increase interactions and produce a fuller understanding.

While the ATS does offer some diagnostic insights, it is not designed for diagnosis. Diagnosis is a multipronged process that utilizes valid assessment instruments (e.g., the Autism Diagnostic Observation Schedule), professional evaluation, and input from teachers and families.

DOI: 10.4324/9781003451266-3

ATS Scale

While ASD is just that, a spectrum, there are phenomena that occur, to different degrees, for individuals on the spectrum. The resulting profile is a description of the individual but also serves as the basis of one's case conceptualization. In this chapter, we will present three individuals, and each case study will be centered on the ATS profile that accompanies this individual. The vast majority of those who are diagnosed with ASD feel separate from the neurotypical community. While there will be connections, such as at school, through special needs activities like sports, and even religious communities, generally, the individual on the autism spectrum is primarily connected to family. Therefore, building additional social outlets is a priority. The ATS allows people to see areas where some type of connection is possible. This chapter will examine three individuals in detail, using the ATS as the primary source of information. These three individuals will span the range of a high-functioning young woman, a mid-functioning young man, and a low-functioning, primarily not-speaking, boy.

The ATS generates a profile of where the individual falls in seven categories. The higher the dot is on the scale, the more functional the individual is in that area. The seven columns examine the following: rigid and repetitive behaviors, sensory concerns, social skills, school/work performance, language, self-regulation, and life skills. Figure 3.1 is an example of an ATS that is blank and has not been filled in to reflect any individual. The ATS is designed to show graphically the issues experienced by the individual on the autism spectrum and the level at which that issue is present.

Column one is the Repetitive and Rigid dimension. As noted on the top of the ATS, this column is the only one that must distinguish whether the behavior noted is internal or external. In other words, snapping one's fingers repeatedly is a repetitive behavior that is external. In contrast, thinking over and over about the size of a dog's teeth, while still a repetitive concern, is internal and not noticed by another person. The scale is designed so that the lower the point on the column, the more disruptive or detrimental that concern is.

The second column focuses on sensory issues. This is an interesting category in that it covers a wide range. In essence, sensory issues of some type are common in the autistic population. However, some sensory issues revolve around avoiding certain sensations (e.g., not being able to tolerate wearing wool), while others are sensory-seeking (e.g., a desire to see a spinning top). This column asks the assessor to determine whether the referenced behavior is disruptive to others or not. Disruptive behavior is rated lower on the column.

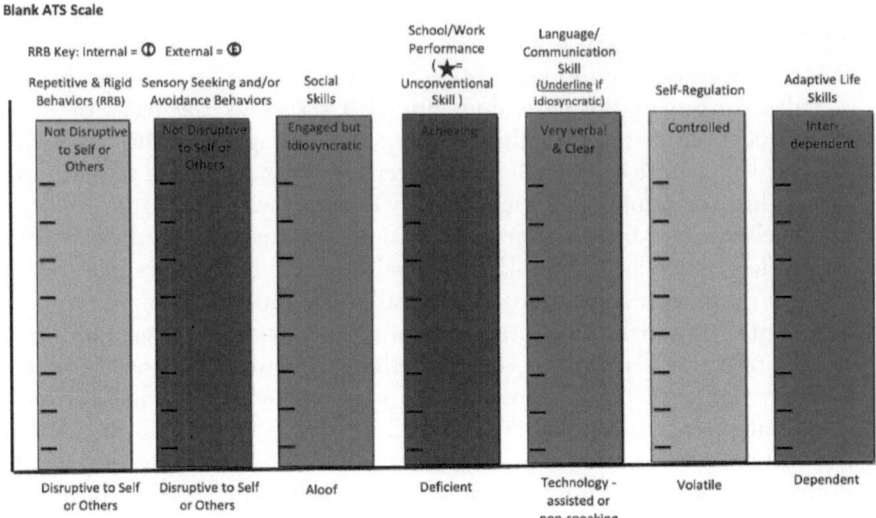

Blank ATS Scale

Figure 3.1 Blank ATS.

The third column is self-explanatory. In essence, the higher the score, the more social the individual. The fourth column is also quite straightforward but adds a unique measure. In short, is the individual able to succeed in a typical classroom? Added into this category is the star, which is meant to denote whether there is a special skill (e.g., the ability to remember movie lines verbatim after seeing a movie once). The fifth column is also very clear. Can the individual use spoken language, and if so, how clearly?

The sixth column is one that is highly relevant to understand since this area can be very dramatic. The area in question is volatility. Does the individual on the autism spectrum regularly lose their temper and present as an annoyance or threat to others? Or does the individual exhibit good self-regulation? And finally, the seventh column. This part of the graph indicates that those who are able to do a great deal for themselves score high, while those who are entirely reliant on others for daily life activities score low in this column.

Three examples will be presented to demonstrate the ATS and its usefulness while assisting those who wish to understand the individual on the autism spectrum and assist in case conceptualization in family treatment.

In other words, the ATS will provide a profile that serves as a shortcut toward envisioning the strengths and challenges of one on the autism spectrum.

ATS Clinical Case: Kayla

This first case, Figure 3.2, represents Kayla, a young woman recently diagnosed who would be considered ASD, Level 1. She attends a typical public school and receives no additional assistance. Her presentation of autism is more connected to her highly focused interests and limited social awareness.

Looking at her profile, one sees that most of the dots fall above the midline of each column, suggesting that while she is on the autism spectrum, the symptoms and related behaviors do not have a paralyzing effect on her day-to-day life. However, it is clear that her internal repetitive and rigid behaviors (which are largely internal) are still somewhat disruptive. For Kayla, her almost constant fascination with the Harry Potter novels and the world constructed for those novels creates an obsessive-like quality to her interest. For Kayla, her enthrallment with all things related to the

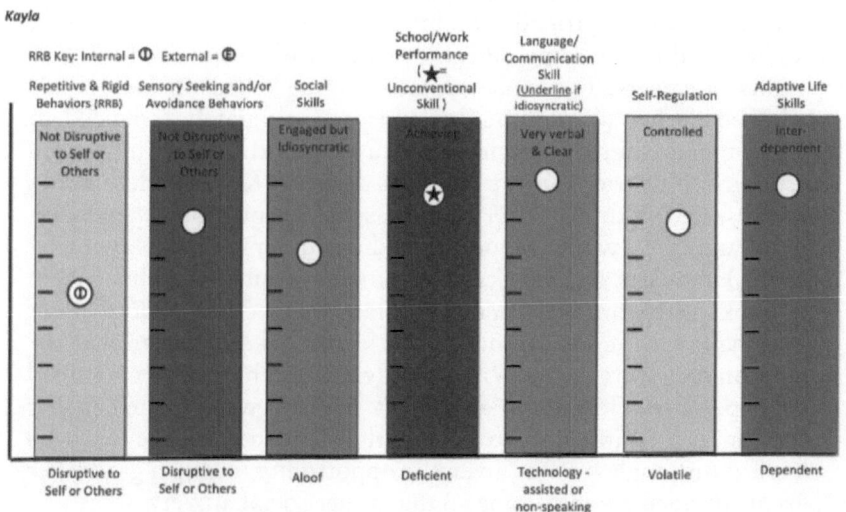

This is intended to be used as a clinical tool only, and is not a research based assessment.
Please place an "s" by any score that is due to a "sensory dysfuncton".

Browning, Manfredi & Abrams 2023

Figure 3.2 High-functioning ATS.

Harry Potter books and movies interferes with her ability to connect naturally with others. This repetitive fascination, while largely going on in her head, causes her to discuss the topic at length, resulting in her being made fun of by her peers. Also, quickly evident is that Kayla is academically strong, has clear communication skills, is self-regulated, and has solid general life skills.

While not a significant problem, her profile would suggest that her desire for sensory stimulation and her social skills are areas in which she struggles a bit and could benefit from treatment. By and large, Kayla's ATS profile is positive, suggesting high intellect, language skills, and the ability to negotiate life skills very well. As the ATS offers only a quick visual snapshot, the case study remains necessary to fully understand the individual on the spectrum.

"High Functioning"– Kayla, cisgender female, age 14; IQ=140

Kayla, age 14, a cisgender female, was diagnosed with autism last year following a depressive episode and a resulting comprehensive psychological evaluation. She began reading independently at age three, to her parents' surprise, and elementary school was a breeze for her academically; she was deemed gifted at age seven. She grew up with a group of friends whom she had known since preschool; they were all in the same playgroup, which was organized by their parents/caregivers. In elementary school, she relied on her friends to introduce her to additional friends and ultimately struggled to maintain many of these friendships. Kayla was known to jump from friend group to friend group out of a desire to feel included. Kayla was obsessed with the Harry Potter series throughout elementary school and often would request that she and her friends play make-believe Hogwarts during recess, where she would recite lines from the books verbatim. Her friends constantly asked her to do this but often made fun of her behind her back; she did not realize that the attention they were giving her was bullying until her teacher confided in her parents. Thinking that Kayla's oddities were related to her superior level of intelligence, they initially brushed off the teacher's worries. Although she was given the opportunity to skip a grade, her parents decided against doing so due to her social anxiety.

Kayla and her group of friends were interspersed between different "teams" during middle school, and Kayla formed new friendships with two groups of females, although she often felt like an outsider. In middle school, a teacher noticed Kayla's knack for English language arts and foreign languages, particularly Spanish. Her teacher offered her the opportunity to go on a student exchange program in Madrid, but after consulting with her parents, she turned down the opportunity due to feeling anxious and worrying that she would not like the food. Kayla is particular about the textures of the foods she eats. Kayla communicated that instead of going to Madrid, she wanted to focus on strengthening her math skills as to prepare for the SATs. Instead, her teacher allowed her to take on an additional foreign language class, Latin. Her parents enrolled her in an after-school math-intensive program. Kayla is now preparing to take her driver's test. Kayla struggled with the transition to high school and found herself lost socially. She began to withdraw more than usual and now procrastinates doing her schoolwork to restart the *Real Housewives* franchise and engage in online chat groups. Kayla often repeats lines from the shows in her mind because it makes her feel good. Kayla was not surprised when she was diagnosed with autism, as she has always felt "different," and is now focused on learning more about her neurotype and connecting with other autistics.

Family: Mother, Mother's boyfriend (not yet introduced to family), Father, Older sister age 23, older brother age 21.

ATS Clinical Case: Ryan

Looking at Figure 3.3, one sees the ATS of Ryan, age 11, who would be considered Level II within the ASD diagnosis. One's eye is drawn to the three lower dots on the first three columns when examining Ryan's ATS. It is in these areas that he is having his greatest difficulties. As you will read, Ryan is clearly on the autism spectrum and is volatile. He is not hurting people, but he does, when frustrated, shove kids and push around furniture. In addition, his big challenges are his difficulty in having a conversation, especially when anxious, and his emotional dysregulation.

When reading the ATS, the therapist generates interventions based on the scale itself. Certain information must be gathered before one can begin to create clinical interventions. Simply having the parents show you where they believe Ryan falls on each dimension creates questions. The therapist does not have to determine why Ryan does what he does. That issue is addressed later in treatment. From the first two columns, it is apparent that Ryan has behaviors and patterns that are disruptive and repetitive. In his case, the clarifying questions would make clear that his dislike of taking a shower due to the discomfort of a wet head, or only drinking

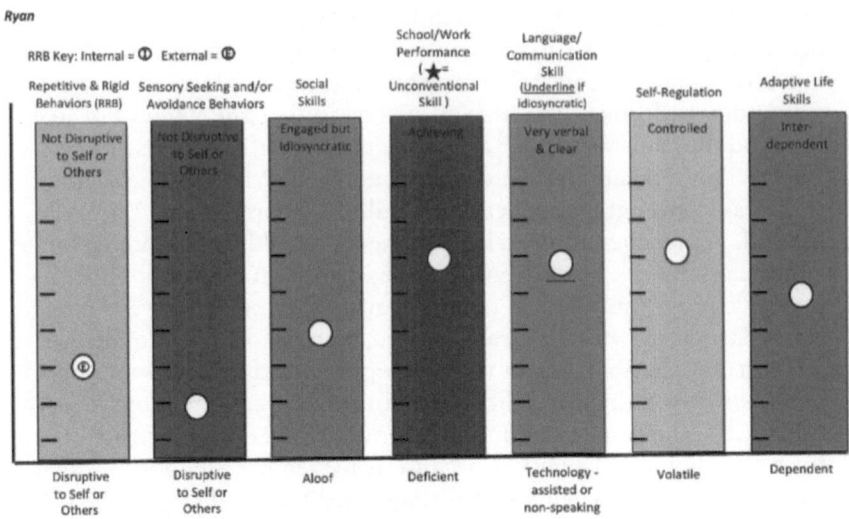

Figure 3.3 Moderate-functioning ATS.

water from a particular bottle are examples of behaviors that, while relatively benign, can cause difficulties for families and teachers.

The very low score on column 2 (Sensory) must be understood carefully. Often, the behavior cannot be fully resolved, so one has to learn to accommodate some behaviors and attempt to reduce or cease others. For Ryan, the intense discomfort with a wet head is problematic for the parents due to an awareness that showers are a common method for bathing, and some cleaning of the hair must occur on occasion. With this knowledge of the difficulty, the therapist, often working with an occupational therapist, finds some alternatives that make this sensitivity less burdensome to both Ryan and his parents.

While Ryan is still challenged with the last four columns (School, Language, Regulation, and Life Skills), these are relative strengths and need to be employed that way. So, the therapist concentrates on moving the dots on the ATS upward. In other words, the ATS provides a road map that one can follow. Improving behaviors mentioned in the first three columns (Rigid/Repetitive, Sensory, Social) at the beginning of treatment is recommended by using the ATS. In a sense, the ATS is a snapshot of the individual at that time. The goal is to raise whatever dots on the columns might indicate improvement in any of the seven areas. Certainly, the profile is difficult to alter since symptoms for individuals on the autism spectrum rarely improve rapidly. However, things often do improve, and one can rescore an ATS after some period of time, often a few years, and improvement will be evident in the revised profile on the new ATS.

"Medium Functioning" – Ryan, cisgender male, age 11, IQ = 99

Ryan, age 11, a cisgender male who has a fraternal twin sister, was diagnosed with autism and attention deficit hyperactivity disorder, combined presentation, when he was six years old. He did not speak in full sentences until he was four years old and struggled with fine and gross motor skills and with maintaining eye contact. He was enrolled in speech and occupational therapies starting at age three, and in early intervention services. Ryan always relied on his sister socially; he felt more comfortable playing with females rather than males due to struggling with coordination and thus not being athletic. Ever since childhood, he has struggled with falling and staying asleep, much to his parents' dismay. Ryan's Individualized Education Plan (IEP) was initiated when he was in the first grade, and he has made significant academic improvements with the support and accommodations he has received to this point. Due to struggling with conversational reciprocity, especially when he is anxious, his sister often initiates conversations when in large groups with other peers. Ryan does not need his sister's help when he is with familiar individuals in small groups.

Ryan's mother and special education teacher constantly remind him to use the restroom and drink water; he will only drink Poland Spring water from a particular plastic bottle. He will not eat foods that are green and will only use plastic utensils because he does not like how metal feels in his mouth. Showering is a constant fight between Ryan and his parents, as he dislikes his hair feeling wet.

In the sixth grade, Ryan is enrolled in an inclusion classroom but spends about a quarter of his school day in a special education classroom. When he becomes stressed or emotional, he struggles to express himself verbally and tends to resort to behavioral aggression. He has made much progress over the past two years and has not been aggressive with anyone in over six months. Ryan's mother believes that the psychotherapy they initiated during the fourth grade has significantly helped him with emotional regulation. Ryan is now able to identify and express his emotions before he gets too emotional, and he asks to use his weighted vest to calm him. His peers have made fun of him for not being able to sit still due to often shaking his leg and blinking, but his stimulating behaviors do not have much of an impact on his functioning; they help him focus. His teacher recently moved Ryan's seat to a higher desk so that he would not bang on the top and disrupt the class. Ryan has recently become close with a female peer in the inclusion class, and they have plans to begin a Pokémon club at school. Ryan yearns to go to college to become a "gamer."

ATS Clinical Case: Max

Finally, Figure 3.4 details an individual, Max, on the low-functioning end of the autism spectrum, diagnosed as Level III in the *DSM-5*.

As will be evident in reviewing Max's ATS, not only is he challenged by significant symptoms of his autism diagnosis, but he is also intellectually

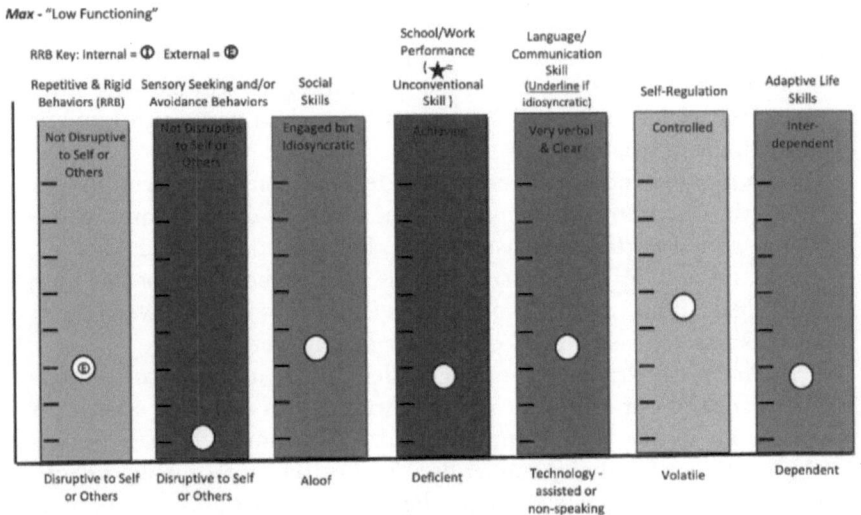

Figure 3.4 Low-functioning ATS.

challenged as well. Between his significant language difficulties, tantrums, and sensory obsessions, Max is someone in need of significant assistance in order to function in school or other settings. He will only wear certain clothing, he constantly desires to chew on something, and he has a highly restricted diet of his own choosing.

In many ways, lower-functioning individuals are somewhat invisible. Due to various factors, these individuals are more likely to be in group homes, and even when they are not, the lack of spoken language makes relational connections more challenging. The ATS highlights that Max has a number of areas that present a challenge to both himself and his family. Both his behaviors and sensory-seeking patterns are disruptive to others, which puts them low on the first two columns. In this case, Max's ATS suggests that not only are his points on the columns low, but there is no area that represents a great strength. This does not mean he has no strengths, but his strengths are relative, and for Max, many areas present a difficulty. One relative strength is that Max is able to communicate somewhat with the use of PECS (picture exchange communication system). Certainly, any improvement in Max being understood by a wider circle of people and any decrease in his sensory-seeking behavior would assist him and his family. While it is unmistakable that Max is low functioning on the autism spectrum, the ATS provides some guidance on understanding his particular challenges. The additional challenges of Max's tendency to elope and his lack of toilet training are significant challenges that will need to be understood and hopefully addressed with either outside support or treatments that can assist in these life-altering areas.

"Low Functioning" – Max, cisgender male, age 13; IQ = 65 -ID

Max, age 13, was diagnosed with autism at age three after his parents and pediatrician noticed that he would not respond to his name when called verbally, was constantly putting objects into his mouth, made humming noises, and often eloped. Ever since he was about four years old, he has refused to wear anything other than SpongeBob T-shirts and gray sweatpants. After enrolling him in early intervention and speech therapy, it was determined that he would benefit from a PECS board to communicate, and a year later, after mastering the use of the device, he transitioned to using Proloquo2Go on an iPad. Though he used to struggle to calm himself when becoming frustrated, which would often result in at least two tantrums daily, his use of the Proloquo2Go has streamlined the communication of his needs and wants. However, he does become emotionally explosive when denied his favorite food, Goldfish crackers, or when he is unable to ride the swings outdoors due to poor weather.

Max spends about 90% of his school day in an autistic support classroom. He tends to follow a male peer in his classroom, but rather than playing together, he will try to take his peers' toys. He does not show much interest in social relationships and will often ignore peers' attempts to initiate collaborative play. Max is constantly chewing on the chewelry his parents purchased for him, as he was previously mouthing pencils and inedible objects. He is fond of his 1:1 aid in the autistic support classroom and often strokes her velvet notebook. Max has recently joined an autistic support group in the community and joins their weekly events with his parents or a direct support professional, as he is not toilet trained and continues to elope often.

Using the ATS in Treatment and School Meetings

As can be seen from this use of the ATS, far greater details are available than simply referring to the level of functioning. The family therapist is advised to use the ATS as a tool to share with the whole family, as well as aides, school personnel, and medical professionals. The ATS should be shared with the grandparents. The more one understands the individual on the autism spectrum, the easier it is to form a relationship. One could speculate that the greatest factor stopping people from forming a relationship with someone with autism is discomfort. It is uncomfortable when one does not know what to say or how to react to the other person. By "reading" the ATS, one is able to see the nuances of ASD in a clearer manner and discuss these issues in a less emotional manner since it is really the ATS that is the centerpiece of the discussion. While one does not want to distance themselves too far from the individual, having the scale provide a foundation for the treatment and education agendas to emerge is helpful.

Examining the ATS in Treatment

In each of the three cases just discussed, the ATS would serve a purpose in treatment. In all three examples, the creation of the ATS with the parents serves the goal of allowing the therapist to observe how the family discusses their child's autism, how closely they agree with each other on the symptoms and strengths, and which areas are presenting significant concerns. The therapist should attend to any area in which the parents are not in agreement regarding their child. For example, on occasion, the mother may be the target of some aggression by a child on the spectrum, whereas the father might be bigger, stronger, and not seen by the child as someone who can be attacked or pushed around. If the couple recognizes this pattern, the father can be supportive of his spouse and serve as a protector, to some extent. However, at times, the father may deny the behavior, having not experienced it, leaving the wife/mother to feel more vulnerable. This can be an important topic since the father might interpret the difference as an indication of his wife doing something to encourage aggression, when usually this difference is simply a matter of the child venting anger at someone they feel is closer to their own strength.

In Kayla's situation, the therapy offered would be to shift her to topics outside of Harry Potter on occasion, as well as to find situations in which her great knowledge about Harry Potter books and movies can be celebrated with like-minded people. It may be worthwhile for Kayla to be referred to a group that is populated with others who are very high functioning, as she is, but also on the autism spectrum. In many ways, trying to make one's social life entirely with neurotypical people can be challenging for one on the autism spectrum and leads many to feel they need to camouflage their own way of seeing the world, leading some to feel bad about themselves.

Moving on to treatment issues with Ryan, there are a few areas that need to be addressed to improve his life, his parents' lives, and his school success. Among the areas that need to be addressed is increasing Ryan's comfort with conversing with others. Again, linking him to a social skills group that is geared toward others, similar to Ryan, increases the likelihood that he will make real friends and find a way to converse without the assistance of his sister. While his sister's help should be acknowledged, it will be critical for Ryan to gain comfort in speaking to others without coaching.

With the consultation of an occupational therapist, the issue of drinking out of a particular bottle can be examined. Is there something about how this bottle works that comforts Ryan? If so, might there be other methods of drinking that can be made appealing? Regarding the plastic utensils, the initial answer might be to let this one go and allow Ryan to use the utensils he prefers. The feel and sound of metal utensils are quite distinct, and pushing Ryan to adjust might not be worth the battle that ensues.

The Extended Family

The extended family is invited to a session. At this session, Beth explains her son, Ryan, to her father, Thomas. While Susan does not speak in this short example, she is Beth's mother. The reference to Bill refers to Ryan's father, and Beth's husband. The ATS serves as a tool that allows a discussion of Ryan in a less emotional manner. (Ryan-child, Beth-Ryan's mother, Bill-Ryan's father, Thomas-Beth's father, Susan-Beth's mother)

Therapist: Thank you, Beth, Susan, and Thomas, for coming to this meeting. I will let your daughter run the show from here. I will interject at certain times.

Beth: Okay, I made copies of our ATS scales for everyone. Let's go to column 1. I placed my dot where I did because I think that his obsession with food color and utensils seems to really get on people's nerves. But, to be clear, it doesn't bother me that much, but I know it makes it hard for others.

Therapist: Yeah, one of the beautiful aspects of family is the acceptance that can occur. When it works well, the families are generally much happier.

Thomas: Even if we get much better at this, aren't there times when he should leave? When he is just too upset?

Beth: That is exactly why I did not want this meeting.

Therapist: No, it is okay. Everyone needs to set their limit. That is how this works. I believe that it will not be needed by your dad at some point, but he needs that.

Therapist: Okay, what is the part of the ATS where Susan and Thomas could learn how to enjoy Ryan more?

Beth: Yeah, really listen to him about Pokémon and ask a couple of real questions.

Thomas: I don't know it well enough, and it is just not fun for me.

Therapist: Here is where we need to all become scholars, Ryan Scholars. We need to reach the place wherein we understand why he just said what he said, even if it is strange, by neurotypical standards. In a sense, it is helpful to recognize that someone on the autism spectrum represents a different culture. For example, if you were to have a Tibetan monk move into your home, and he followed his typical day, you would be a bit puzzled, annoyed by, curious, understanding, and happy. In a similar way, this is what happens in the family on the autism spectrum (FotAS). Beth and Bill have become total Ryan Scholars. They understand, to some extent, why he does what he does. That level of understanding derives from proximity, not brilliance. The grandparents, aunts, and uncles are a step removed. They generally see Ryan at family gatherings and thus have limited opportunities to understand fully the reasons for some of his actions and comments.

Returning to the example with the monk, Bill and Beth, being the people who live in the home the monk lives in, would need to explain what this monk does. We are not surprised by exact instructions (e.g., "Tibetan monks pray multiple times a day"), and this level of explanatory detail is not perceived as overly informative. But if a family member explains their child in great detail, it is often perceived as a challenge to the other person that they are not being a good relative or family member. The fact that autism creates a unique culture is often lost, so coaching others on how to respond to someone on the autism spectrum is often interpreted in a negative way. Therapists need to assist family members in discussing the child on the autism spectrum in a manner that suggests that the child represents a unique culture so that questions and explanations become natural and supportive. Certainly, no parent is absolutely certain about every action and reaction by their child on the autism spectrum, but they are far more informed and aware than others.

Examining the ATS in School IEP Meetings

The ATS serves as a tremendous tool for families attempting to educate school districts as to the areas of strength and challenges of their children on the autism spectrum. Often, school meetings can drift into an adversarial posture between the school personnel and the family of one on the spectrum. Systemic factors, sometimes financial, can affect the capacity to work as a team. Moving the meeting toward a more factual stance often cuts some of the tension in the meeting. The ATS provides that tool. Family members, the child themselves, school personnel, and psychotherapists all use the same tool. By looking at each other's scoring of the ATS, areas of agreement and potential disagreement can be discussed.

Using Collaborative Problem-solving when the Problem is Tantrums

An important adjunct treatment will be teaching the parents and teachers the Collaborative Problem Solving (CPS) method developed by Ross Greene (Greene & Ablon, 2006). CPS is a method that takes the position that for some children, simple discipline, such as saying "no" to the child, backfires since some children (and certainly children on the autism spectrum in many cases) are unable to interpret why they need to do certain things (e.g., go to the doctor, tolerate loud noises, do homework before playing) that are treated as important, and the insistence by a parent or teacher, without understanding the child's reluctance, results in tantrums. Greene speculates that tantrums, which he terms "explosions," only generate additional explosions. Thus, a system is needed that allows the child to be heard, understood, and respected. Only then is the child confronted with the fact that the request by the adult needs to be addressed, thus leading to a pattern of working together to solve the issue confronting both the child and the adult. The term "Collaborative Problem Solving" is the method embraced, and such efforts can often lessen tantrums (Greene & Ablon, 2006).

For example, in the example of Ryan, the school needs to embrace some version of CPS, but the school is right, to some extent, that this is a challenge for teachers. CPS seems to take more time. The time is up front. Learning how to move off of insisting on an action (e.g., "get down to dinner right now") to accepting that some children need to be understood before they can accept correction is a necessary step in addressing children prone to moving into a tantrum. In other words, when a child has an area of difficulty (e.g., great difficulty in transitioning), the pushing of the agenda only causes the child to become overwhelmed and thus go into a tantrum. Often, children on the autism spectrum meet this criterion.

Ryan, in conjunction with his parents, has responded well to CPS; therefore, the home is getting more stable. Tantrums are far fewer. The problem is that Ryan's teachers believe that, in many cases, using CPS takes longer than other methods. However, Greene argues that in the long run, the time to achieve the goal of discipline is shorter with CPS because with the "explosive child," the time lost during tantrums is substantial, and even after the tantrum, these children are often emotionally exhausted.

In addition, the Pathways Inventory, which is a form in the CPS materials, highlights areas of lagging skills, often directly related to the tantrums and outbursts causing concern. If tantrums are the central issue, the CPS method is the priority. If the issue is about autism symptoms more specifically, the ATS form is particularly useful. For example, Ryan does have significant tantrums. So, while the ATS assists those in the IEP meeting in understanding Ryan's autism style, the Pathways Inventory is particularly useful for lessening tantrums.

The following is a clinical example of the school psychologist and the parent advocating the **CPS approach to the teacher in an IEP meeting.**

Parent:	We were hoping that the CPS method could be used with Ryan in the class.
Teacher:	Well, when Ryan starts to get upset, it seems too late to follow the Collaborative Problem Solving technique of empathy, defining the problem, and invitation to collaborate.
School Psychologist:	That is true; it is better to know what Ryan's triggers are before they are set off. Let's look at his Pathways Inventory. Clearly, transitions are difficult for Ryan, and most tantrums are connected to some type of transition.

Teacher:	You mean I need to prepare him for transitions? I have 28 kids.
School Psychologist:	It actually is helpful for the whole group. Just increasing preparation. "We will be leaving in five minutes." Short, clear statements about what is happening can be very useful. If you feel the class would feel patronized by this, just mention it to Ryan. The class knows he needs assistance. Ryan does not enjoy having tantrums.
Parent:	It is really true. The CPS method is really working at home.
Teacher:	So, I would just say, toward Ryan, "lunch in 5 minutes."
School Psychologist:	That is what we would like to start with.
Teacher:	Okay, I am glad to try that. But Ryan has to able to calm down enough to not disturb the class.
Parent:	We can assure you, he can be calmed down pretty fast, but you need to get why he freaking out. Usually, Ryan does not understand why he is upset.
Teacher:	We need you to help us at home by clarifying to him what he needs to do.
Parent:	Okay, we will. Let us know what you want. But we need to know you are trying to understand that he needs someone to confirm what is bothering him. It is unfortunate that this is a challenge for Ryan, but it is. The good news is he able to calm down much better at home now. We have totally changed how we talk when he is about to tantrum. I am glad to give an example, if helpful.
School:	Sure, how would you handle when he starts to scream about needing a different color bottle in the cafeteria?
Parents:	You quietly look him in the eye and say, "It really upsets you to not have your green bottle." After he agrees with that statement, we say, "Since your green bottle was dirty before and needed to be washed, do you have any ideas about getting something to drink?"

The IEP meeting continues, but whenever the parent feels that alerting the school personnel to a feature of Ryan's behavior is necessary, the ATS can be returned to as a tool to increase and clarify how Ryan is perceived.

Using the ATS in an IEP Meeting

The ATS is filled out by the parents, and copies are made for the participants of the IEP. Certainly, if the school personnel wish to contest or edit the

ATS, that is fine. The instrument is a working document that is meant to be edited with improvements or backsliding being reflected.

The following is an example of how the ATS may be useful in an IEP meeting.

Parent: I think if you look at Ryan's ATS, you will see the dot in the language column in the middle. While we know that his language remains a concern, we have been impressed when he gets a little angry at his sister when she picks up and speaks for him. He has gotten much more confident and challenges her not to speak for him as much.

Teacher: I am not sure how that is relevant since Sally is in the other class.

Parent: Yes, we know, but it suggests to us that expecting Ryan to be able to answer may be improving.

Teacher: But I thought we were going to try not to frustrate him.

Parent: We think that if there was a way to know if he knew the answer, like if he looked directly at you during a class discussion, he might be ready to be a little more involved.

Conclusion

The Autism Trait Scale (ATS) is a tool that assists one in creating a graphic profile of one on the autism spectrum. The ATS is useful when working with a family, the school, a congregation, and professionals. The graph is filled out by some of those using the tool, while others are just looking at it and listening to the opinions of those who know the individual on the autism spectrum well. No one has to agree with every rating. There is no "correct" rating. Each rating is interpreted, at some level, by the person filling in the scale itself. For example, some symptoms really annoy one person, and the other is not as frustrated by the behavior. A wife may feel that hearing about Beauty and the Beast, for the four hundredth time (determining if Gaston is evil, or foolish) is a topic she does not mind, since it makes her feel close to her daughter. Yet, her husband, who does love their child, finds this topic totally unhelpful and wants the discussion to stop. On the first column, they will score their daughter very differently. The wife places her dot (as both internal and external) above the midline of the column. The husband (father) places his dot (labeling it as only external) well below the midline. They both know their daughter very well, but they see this behavior from a different perspective from one another. Since there is no right answer to the placement of a dot on the ATS, it is a point of discussion. The wife must consider whether it is time to agree with her husband and shut down the discussion regarding Gaston as an unhelpful obsession. Or, the father might come to believe that since their daughter is not bringing the topic up often outside the home, it really is a consuming interest, and if his wife wishes to engage her daughter on this topic in order to comfort their daughter, there is no great harm.

The therapist uses this material to help the family members understand their positions better and hopefully work together as good partners. As has been mentioned in this chapter, this work is intended to help family members work together, and incorporate other people (teachers, doctors, community members) into a team, understanding the individual on the autism spectrum. This process is intended to make people on the autism spectrum proud of themselves and understood by others.

Note

1   I wish to thank Zoey Abrams for graphic assistance on the three ATS scales and for creating the case studies.

References

American Psychiatric Association. (2013). *Diagnostic and statistical manual of mental disorders* (5th ed.). https://doi.org/10.1176/appi.books.9780890425787

Green, R., & Ablon, J. S. (2006). *Treating explosive kids: The collaborative problem-solving approach*. New York, NY: The Guilford Press.

4 Early Diagnosis, Clinical Concerns, and the School System

"What to Expect" and Navigating the School Systems and Assessments

Britney Fontes and Gwendolyn Edwards

How Early can Someone be Diagnosed with Autism?

One study by Howlin and Asgharian found that out of 770 families, about half of them could see signs of autism in their children as early as two years old, and about 93 percent reported they could notice features as early as three years old, although a diagnosis is not typically given until about age 11 (1997; Howlin and Asgharian, 1999). Usually, when a parent, teacher, or close family friend notices signs that something does not seem right or is different about a young child, the first thing someone does is go to their medical provider. A provider will likely conduct an informal assessment, also known as a screener, and ask several questions about the child's social, emotional, cognitive, relational, and physical development. A screener should also provide some insight into the genetic risks of a child having autism, such as if there is a family or sibling history of autism. In any case, medical physicians are not necessarily experts in diagnosing autism, and it is best if parental guardians can seek a formal neurocognitive assessment to explore whether there are any further concerns or questions. It may also be the case that at first, a child may appear to be developing typically compared to their peers and does not present with significant atypicality, thus being turned away by doctors with no concerns. The family may later find that at age six, their child does, in fact, meet the criteria for autism. This means that if doctors dismiss families at first, but years later, their child's development still appears concerning, families should continue to seek an updated assessment and support.

Stats/Research

In one fascinating study that followed 20 families, researchers found that children who went through an extensive autism assessment and received a diagnosis at the age of two still maintained reliable diagnosis at a two- to three-year follow-up (More & Goodson, 2003). Although some

DOI: 10.4324/9781003451266-4

presentations of autism may vary from person to person, the general rule of thumb is to identify autism as soon as possible to ensure the earliest forms of interventions. The earlier a family can receive support, the better off they may be in understanding their child, finding unique pathways toward success, and building a supportive community. Identifying autism early also allows families and the educational system to appropriately adapt to the child's underlying cognitive issues sooner rather than later, which has been discussed intensively in research showing that early detection followed by intervention can be crucial to a child's success (Corsello, 2005; Fenrell et al., 2013). It should also be noted that if a child received an early atypical autism diagnosis or a pervasive developmental disorder not otherwise specified, their symptoms could change over time. This would require an ongoing assessment to ensure an accurate diagnosis. In other words, the presentation of autism tends to be stable, long-term, and persistent, whereas other neurodevelopmental disorders can change (Rondeau et al., 2011; Fernell et al., 2013).

Autism and Divorce

When a couple decides to start a family, they will face many challenges and new experiences, some of which they may be prepared for and many of which (like most parenting) can be an exciting and daunting experience. Feelings surrounding new parenthood are typical and expected but nonetheless can be overwhelming and scary. When an infant enters the world, the couple has to adjust every aspect of their life to care for and accommodate a tiny human while balancing their roles from being a partner to a parent. Inevitably, the birth of a child places the couple's overall wellbeing on the back burner. So, how does this already profound experience change when a child has autism? To be clear, the majority of families, regardless of disability, will go through developmental growing pains and joyful celebrations. However, having a child with a disability can affect how milestones and "typical developmental stages" are experienced. For example, a child with autism who is nonverbal may not be starting preschool or kindergarten with same-age peers, or they may be late to being potty trained, which in some cases can limit a family's access to childcare if a facility requires children to be able to use the bathroom by themselves. This can leave parents to have feelings of fear or sadness about their child missing out on different social aspects of school, feeling as though they did not "do enough" during developmental periods, or that they "did something wrong," all of which are typical reactions. Fast-forward to early adulthood, when children typically leave home, otherwise known as "launching." Parents may have adult children who live in the home longer than expected, which can affect parents' experience of "the empty nest," thus influencing their ability to reconnect as a couple.

Parenting a child with autism can pose many challenges, including stress on the marriage (Setltzer et al., 2000). Hartley and colleagues conducted a profound research study that examined 391 parents of children with autism over several decades using previously recorded data, interviews, and public divorce data. Interestingly, when compared to 391 parents of children who did not have a disability, parents of autism had a divorce rate (23.13%) almost twice as high as the control group (13.81%) (Hartley et al., 2010). However, it should be noted that in the study, three-fourths of the parents of autistic children did remain together despite the challenges of autism spectrum disorder (ASD). In other words, although parents of autism are more likely to get divorced than families who do not have a child with autism, the percentage is fairly low. Still, one should consider the possible variables contributing to families of autism having more difficulty with marriage. One reason may be that parents give one another less attention due to the increased attention that may be necessary to care for a child with specific needs. In addition to couples attempting to meet their spouse's needs, parents may also experience increased parental stress. Naseef and Freedman, who are experts in autism and family research, say that parents do not have enough time to attend to the marriage and spend additional effort on one another, which can be exacerbated by being physically and emotionally overwhelmed (2012).

Researchers also found that families of autism were at a higher risk of divorce for a longer period of time compared to parents without a child with autism (Hartley et al., 2010). Researchers also found that families of autism were at a higher risk of divorce for a longer period of time compared to parents without a child with autism. Similarly to previous myths that that families of autism have an 80% risk of divorce, although there is little evidence to support this claim. In, fact this is not true when controlling for relevant covariates" (Freedman et al., 2012). In fact, that is not true. Naseef and Freedman (2012) support the notion that families are making the decision to stay together more often than originally believed by mainstream media. Similar to the divorce study, Freedman et al. (2012) explored the rate at which children with autism continue to live with their parents. Although the researchers did not exclusively look at divorce rates, 64% of the families in their study remained intact.

What Does this Mean for Families of Autism?

When clinicians are providing an autism diagnosis to families for the first time, it is essential that they meet with both parental figures. Even if the parents are not romantically together but share custody or caregiver responsibilities, clinicians need to make their best effort to include each parent in treatment. Of course, not all families are what we once knew as "traditional" and may comprise various structures, including extended, blended, and multigenerational families. For the purpose of this chapter, the primary focus will be on married parents. While much of this information will be relevant to a wider parental population, it is important to be respectful of the limitations of the research. Parents of those on the autism spectrum need to know that receiving an autism diagnosis can result in additional burdens on the relationship that they may not have previously considered when deciding to start a family. For example, raising a child or children with autism can be mentally, emotionally, and financially taxing, which can ultimately drain each parent, making parents more prone to burnout and stress. Families need to be aware of this reality because parents are the foundation of a child's well-being and long-term development. If parents face challenges with communication, with finding time for one another, and with healthy coping, they could experience a greater chance of divorce, ultimately affecting family dynamics and the child's well-being. All new parents need to be aware that their dynamics as a couple may shift, though parents of autism need to make an extra effort to maintain a strong relationship. Naseef and Freedman (2012) found that mothers' parenting stress was associated with fathers' positive experiences of their children. This may suggest that parental perception of parenting can influence a partner's experience of positive or negative beliefs. In other words, a father's experience of parenting stress may also directly impact a mother's mental health and experience of stress. This notion speaks to the fact that in family systems, each member has an influence on the other person, and relationships are bidirectional. If a father is struggling to manage his child on the spectrum, a mother might indirectly feel this stress and be burdened by disappointment and frustration. Similarly, if a mother is able to find positive aspects of their child with autism, a father may be able to have a more positive experience of parenting, thus allowing the mother to feel relief and support.

Family Therapy

When parents are seeking therapeutic support, it is important that mental health professionals meet with the parents alone and ask what they imagined their life would be like having their first child or growing their family by having additional children. Clinicians need to inquire about the beliefs and fantasies that families imagined for themselves and the entire family system. The family system may go beyond parents and their children and also include grandparents, aunts, uncles, and cousins, who may have a consistent and significant influence on the family. This is essential not only to get a sense of which ideals may need to be revisited but also which dreams can still exist and have reasonable potential. For example, a parent may envision their child getting married one day and suddenly be filled with panic that it is no longer possible upon hearing the news that their child has autism. However, marriage may still be possible, and this fear should be discussed by an expert through psychoeducation, if applicable. In the same light, if parents are informed that their child is quite low functioning, they may need additional time and space to grieve as well as adapt their ideas of the life their child could have had. Parents should be treated through an empathic, nonjudgmental approach, allowing them to feel frustration, sadness, guilt, and remorse. Instead of families holding onto complicated feelings and repressing frustration, parents need the space to share their initial reactions. Since parenting is a bidirectional relationship, both parents must be seen together to explore how each person is experiencing and understanding one another and directly share what they want and need. Regardless of family makeup, raising a child with autism requires additional effort to practice patience, communication, and flexibility. Some parents may be wondering how any of this is even possible when one might be exhausted and feel like there is not a second in the day to connect as a couple. Naseef and Freedman (2012) make a few suggestions that suggest doing the best you can in the face of life's challenges. For example, parents can stay up after the kids are asleep, socialize with friends even if the kids are around, take a break from talking about autism, and take a short walk around the neighborhood. Some families should be encouraged to utilize grandparents and other extended family members to ease parental duties and allow couples time to take a break. Grandparents especially may find a sense of purpose and identity in helping care for a grandchild, thus positively affecting their child as well. If grandparents play a vital role in the family system, they should also be included in family therapy or, at the very least, in discussions around school services. The goal is that everyone is on the same page when it comes to understanding what accommodations a child may need and how the family is going to work together to achieve optimal communication and support. Parents should also be offered ongoing treatment to manage the ups and downs of raising a child with autism, especially as it relates to the relationship of the caregivers. Similarly, if grandparents partake in additional parental roles, they should have the option to meet with a mental health professional to address any concerns around burden, frustration, questions around autism, and family system concerns.

Culture Matters

The best therapeutic practice has mental health providers consider each family's faith and cultural factors and how families understand mental health, mental health treatment, disabilities, and diagnosis. The purpose of exploring cultural factors is to consider beliefs, values, and ideas about why and how things come to be. Mental health professionals may need to provide additional psychoeducation regarding biology, genetics, and neuroscience that accurately describes autism and its biological attributes. Clinicians may need to be mindful of the incorporation of using faith as a positive coping mechanism in families where it is appropriate to do so. Cultural factors and beliefs may also shed light on how families may internalize and experience the diagnosis of autism. Suppose a parent experiences shame about the diagnosis of autism or identifies with various minority groups. In that case, they may be less likely to ask for help due to stigma, discrimination, or healthy cultural mistrust. Similarly, if a father is less emotional due to certain stereotypes that some societies project onto men, he may be hesitant to share if he is struggling with parenting a child with autism. In other words, a father may feel additional pressure to be strong and not falter in the face of challenges. Clinicians need to understand how parents cope as individuals and as a couple to promote healthy adaptive functioning and growth as a family.

A Child is Ready for School—What Happens Now?

The summer starts to wind down, and all the "Back to School" sales begin. For some parents, reminders like the end of summer may be harmless or exciting, and for others, it could cause feelings of dread. There are many questions and stressors that may arise for parents when starting school for their child(ren) with autism, such as worrying whether their child is "having a good day" with behaviors, having open communication with the school, and trusting that their child will share information when they get home. Additional concerns include a child being in a new environment and transitioning to different subjects or classes, using transportation, riding the bus for the first time, and so on. The list can go on. As we know, children can feed off our energy. The nervous energy that accompanies any big milestone, like the first day of school or a new school, can create anxiety in parents. A parent being anxious about a child starting school is completely valid but ultimately can make the child more anxious or nervous. If caregivers can provide a calm environment while validating the child's fears as they arise, this could be a way to provide a safe space for them. Engaging in activities to help parents or caregivers stay positive and calm can be beneficial. Children are often very attuned to parents' behavior and will mirror what parents do and hear. It is important for parents to do their best to stay positive, even if they have valid reasons to worry. Knowing that the adjustment period to a new school and the anxiety and fears that come from this experience are reasonable and typical for parents is important. School can be an unknown territory for the family unit, especially for those with ASD. It is likely that there will be an adjustment period for both the children and parents. It may be helpful, when appropriate, for parents to speak with a child's teachers before the school year begins to establish a line of open communication. Open communication in the school setting can simply be informing the teacher about a child, getting to know them better, or letting teachers know when parents need to be contacted. For example, parents can send a child with a note or send an email sharing all the things they like, dislike, dietary restrictions, or triggers that occur at home, which would be applicable for the classroom, and how to de-escalate the situation. Caregivers should not be afraid to share what their goals and wishes are for the school year! Most teachers will welcome this information, and it might help alleviate concerns on that first day. Parents should also find support, whether that be seeking other parent support groups for children on the spectrum or meeting other parents at school functions. Creating a sense of community can be incredibly powerful for families and can translate as a direct reminder that they are not alone.

Parental Advocacy and Autism: How do Parents Advocate for Their Child?

Children with autism require access to a range of health and educational services and supports, and one avenue for accommodations is in the school setting. Parents are often the primary advocates for their children across various programs, which can cause them to report their children's health conditions to professionals in hopes of receiving access to appropriate services. Children with autism often have additional diagnoses (also labeled as "co-morbidities"), such as attention deficit hyperactivity disorder (ADHD), seizure disorders, anxiety, and gastrointestinal disorders. Therefore, advocating for needs that accurately cover the scope of everything that the child may need to be successful may seem daunting or intimidating. The remainder of this chapter is aimed at instilling hope and confidence and normalizing this process so that parents and caregivers can be equipped to advocate for their children.

Parents of children with autism are faced with many challenges. One study found that having a child with ASD resulted in parents experiencing a sense of isolation because of a perceived lack of understanding from society and unsupportive systems (Woodgate et al., 2008). Results indicated that experts and professionals did not always have the necessary knowledge and expertise to navigate the needs of families who have family members with autism. These deficits in understanding, knowledge, and expertise can understandably cause a parent stress and to push for the appropriate care for their child in any setting and to be able to advocate for that care. Researchers describe advocacy as any action taken by a parent on behalf of their child or other children with autism to ensure adequate support, proper level of care, and basic human rights (Ewles, Clifford & Minnes, 2014; Goldman et al., 2020).

Nevertheless, parents are sometimes reluctant and intimidated to advocate in the school system for their child with ASD because they feel as though they lack essential knowledge of the education process. This may be the time when they often request support from a special education advocate when it is available to them. In the United States, parents of children with ASD are more than ten times more likely to pursue legal advocacy when compared to groups in other disability categories. Some scholars argue that this is due in part to the public and private school systems' limited success in effectively and efficiently addressing this complex disability (Zirkel, 2011; Goldman et al., 2020).

Advocacy is an active process that changes depending on the circumstances and needs of the child and parent or caregiver. Parents and caregivers are considered to be natural advocates due to their implicit commitment to the well-being of their children. However, many parents view advocacy as a moral obligation or expectation, and not all parents and guardians are able to effectively advocate for a child with ASD. Advocacy can be a coping strategy for parents of children with disabilities, but too much of this may not be beneficial to the child or the parent. There is some debate about whether parents sometimes intervene too much on their child's behalf (Ewles et al., 2014). Therefore, it is important, like many things in life, to do things in moderation and balance other coping mechanisms, for example, finding support from other individuals who are also going through similar situations and not fully relying on just advocacy work as an aspect of parental identity. Advocacy skills for parents of children with autism may include understanding ASD, using clear and effective communication, being organized, and managing difficult situations when they arise. Several contextual factors may increase or decrease parental advocacy over time, such as financial status, education and skills, time commitment, the severity of the child's condition, and the age of diagnosis (Goldman et al., 2020).

Seeking Help with Assessment and Diagnosis in the School Setting

The following is directly addressed to parents and caregivers of children with autism. Have you ever wondered, if a child does not already have an ASD diagnosis, how you go about getting them diagnosed? The assessment and diagnosis process will be covered in Chapter 5 more thoroughly, although we will begin to lay out the groundwork here. As discussed earlier in this chapter, the child's pediatrician may be the first place to start to get a referral regarding neurodivergent behaviors you may be noticing at a young age through discussing different symptoms and screeners. Advocating for screenings and assessments may be the first time you discuss your child's needs and symptoms that you have noticed and experienced over their developmental periods. Another possibility is that maybe your child met all developmental milestones and did not show any of the typical diagnostic "red flags," but then started school and is struggling with peers, teachers, and classes. As a parent, no one wants to watch their child struggle, and one can feel helpless trying to figure out how to get services for children so that they can succeed socially and academically.

The first thing to know and remember is that your child has the right to a free and appropriate education. The Individuals with Disabilities Education Act (IDEA), which was first enacted in 1975 and revised in 2004, mandates that each state provide all eligible children with a public education that meets their individual needs. The Individuals with Disabilities Act (IDEA) was renamed the Individuals with Disabilities Education Improvement Act, but most people still refer to it as the IDEA. The IDEA specifies that children with various disabilities, including autism, are eligible for early intervention services and special education. With the diagnosis of autism, your child should be able to gain access to the rights defined by the IDEA. The IDEA legislation established an important role for parents in their children's education. You, as a parent, are entitled to be treated as an equal partner with the school district in deciding on an education plan for your child and his or her individual needs. You can be a powerful advocate for your child and an active participant in planning and monitoring your child's unique program and legal rights.

Private versus Public

In understanding the IDEA, a key phrase is "public schools." Why is this important? Shouldn't my child receive an education that meets their needs everywhere? Yes, they should be able to have a right to education. However, it is important to know what the services are and how to access them, as public versus private schools will be different. Within public schools, you can request an evaluation (an example of a formal request letter is at the end of this chapter), which then initiates a 60-day timeline for the school to respond to your request by fulfilling the evaluation request or refusing to evaluate your child. If, by chance, the school responds by stating that they refuse to test your child or that your child does not qualify for special education, you can fight this decision by requesting mediation. Mediation is a voluntary process aimed at establishing agreement between parents and administrators. If mediation is unsuccessful, then a due process hearing is a legal proceeding that attempts to resolve the dispute, which may include filing a complaint with the Bureau of Special Education Appeals. However, if you submit a request and then consent to have an evaluation conducted by the school, the evaluation will begin. This should include direct testing of the child and input from the parent and teachers to accurately assess what needs and accommodations the child would need to be successful in that school district.

Private schools can offer special education, but they are not required to do so. If a private school chooses to provide special services, some schools may offer what is often known as an Instructional Services Plan or an Individual Service Plan, both known as ISPs. This happens when a private school works to provide specialized services within its own system. Additionally, if you and your child choose a private school, they will most likely get a *service plan* through your local education agency (LEA)—not through the private school itself. The LEA manages services and funding for schools in the local area it covers. "Local" can mean different things in different areas. It is important to understand how each private school defines this, as it could be defined as state, regional, or individual school districts.

Private school students who have been parentally placed do not have the same rights to special education services as public school students. As previously discussed, this could be a very upsetting realization for these parents, who feel as though they must now be educational advocates for their children. As always, it is important to check your state's regulations regarding public versus private school settings as well as IEP and 504 plans because there could be varying information and application of rules across different states. At a minimum, the local school district must be able to provide students who are enrolled in private schools an evaluation upon request to determine whether the student is eligible for special education services. Once eligible, the resident school district must offer a Free Appropriate Public Education (FAPE) in the public school, which ultimately, the parent could refuse and instead decide to place the child in a non-public school setting. For example, say your child is enrolled in Sunnyside Private School, and the child or student is having difficulties in the classroom academically and socially, which has been reported by multiple teachers and is something that you and your partner have also been struggling with at home. However, these behaviors are being brought to your attention, and the question arises, "would this child benefit from being evaluated to understand the reason for these behaviors?" This type of evaluation would need to be completed by a psychologist. Therefore, a parent can submit a formal request for their child to be evaluated by the school, and once the request is submitted, the school district that the child resides in is responsible for the evaluation, not Sunnyside. In this example, the child attending Sunnyside Private School's "local" school district is the Columbia School District, a 30-minute drive from the private school. Following the evaluation by the Columbia School District, that school district would offer a free public education, which the child and parent can accept or deny, but in this way, the criteria for the right to education have been met.

A Child Needs an IEP, But What Is It?

The Individualized Education Plan (IEP) is a plan or program developed to ensure that a child who has a disability identified under the law and is attending an elementary or secondary educational institution, receives specialized instruction and related services. The next chapter will discuss IEP plans and examples more thoroughly, but it is an important topic to define and build upon. Not all students who have disabilities require specialized instruction. An IEP document is created to outline specific accessibility requirements for students with disabilities who do require specialized instruction, or for students with disabilities who do not require specialized instruction but need the assurance that they will receive equal access to public education and services. Students with an IEP should expect this plan to be updated annually to ensure that they receive the most effective accommodations for their specific circumstances, and parents should not be alarmed if they are expected to attend IEP update meetings multiple times a year. These meetings can be incredibly helpful for the parents, the child, the teachers, and anyone else who is a part of their care team to discuss their goals for the year and how the school can support the achievement of those goals.

What's a 504 Plan, and How is it Different from an IEP?

The 504 plan is a plan developed to ensure that a child who has a disability identified under the law and is attending an elementary or secondary educational institution, receives accommodations that will ensure the student's academic success and access to the learning environment. If a child does not qualify for special education services under the IDEA, the child may still qualify to receive services under section 504 if what the child is experiencing is shown to limit and impact his or her educational performance substantially. Section 504 applies when a disability substantially limits a major life function, including learning. When a student is excluded from an activity due to disability, a 504 plan is needed to provide accommodations and support for access to both academic and extracurricular activities. For some parents, a 504 plan can be confusing, and they may wonder how this plan differs from an IEP. A child with a disability that would fall under a 504 plan is one who has a physical or mental impairment that considerably limits major life activities. Examples of this would be: a student breaks their arm in multiple places and cannot write; therefore, the district provides someone to take notes or write the homework; a student is deaf and plays sports and the district provides an interpreter for the classroom and any school sports activities they are involved in; a student has cancer, diabetes, epilepsy, migraines, allergies, or asthma, and they are allowed to obtain treatment or medication, as needed; and a student is under a doctor's care for depression or anxiety, frequent behavioral problems, such as ADHD, and therefore is given additional time for completing assignments and allowed to sit in the front of the classroom. Accommodations often refer to building accessibility, classroom adjustments, and curriculum modifications, and they may be updated or revised as needed. Another question that may arise is: Does ADHD not fall under an IEP? And if my child has both ADHD and ASD, how will that affect their special education plans for school? Chapter 5 will go into more detail about the differences between an IEP and a 504 and how accommodations for each, ASD and ADHD, would be covered in a plan.

Conclusion

Navigating early diagnosis and clinical concerns can be stressful for the entire family system, especially for the parents. New situations such as daycare, playgroups, and school can cause a lot of fear and anxiety of the unknown. Parents' being a calm support for a child can help ease his or her nerves about school and help them advocate for the child's needs. Parental advocacy is a life-long process for parents of children with ASD, and the school setting can be one of the first experiences of advocacy for parents. Advocacy work includes various aspects such as time, financial, and emotional commitments and overall providing a future to make things better for their child as they progress in their ASD journey. A major aspect of advocacy work revolves around advocating for the right to education. Being able to request an evaluation within the school, whether in a private or a public school setting, is one step of that journey. IEPs and 504 plans can be relevant factors for a child receiving accommodations in the classroom to help their educational experience.

SAMPLE LETTER REQUESTING EDUCATIONAL EVALUATION

Today's Date (include month, day, and year)

From: Your Name, address, telephone number

To: Name of Principal/IEP Coordinator, Name of School

Re: Your child's name (DOB)

Dear (Principal's name), My name is (your name) and my child, (child's name), is in the (__) grade in (name of teacher)'s class at (name of school).

I am writing to formally request that (child's name) be evaluated for special education services under the Child Find obligations of the Individuals with Disabilities Education Act (IDEA).

As you may know, my child has been having difficulty with (provide detailed information about your concerns, using supporting evidence such as test scores, teacher communications, work samples, etc.). I have spoken with (name of teacher) about these concerns and the following things have been tried to help.

(Describe any interventions that were tried, including response to intervention [RTI] and informal accommodations in the classroom). I believe it is critical for (child's name) to be evaluated. As part of this process and conversation, I also would like to request that (child's name) be assessed under Section 504 of the Rehabilitation Act of 1973 to see whether (s/he) has a disability as defined by that law.

I understand that you will send me an evaluation plan explaining the tests that may be given to my child. I would also appreciate any other information you have regarding the evaluation process. If you need more information, please contact me at (your phone number).

Thank you very much for your help. I look forward to hearing from you soon.

Sincerely,
Your name

Copy sent to:
your child's teacher
your child's education record

---

*Adapted from The Everything Parent's Guide to Special Education (Adams Media, 2014)

References

Corsello, C. (2005). Early intervention in autism. Infants & young children. *Journal of Infants and Young Children, 18*(2), 74–85.

Ewles, G., Clifford, T., & Minnes, P. (2014). Predictors of advocacy in parents of children with autism spectrum disorders. *Journal of Developmental Disabilities, 20*, 73–82.

Goldman, S. E., Burke, M. M., Casale, E. G., Frazier, M. A., & Hodapp, R. M. (2020). Families requesting advocates for children with disabilities: The who, what, when, where, why, and how of special education advocacy. *Intellectual and Developmental Disabilities, 58*(2), 158–169. doi:10.1352/1934-9556-58.2.158

Hartley, S. L., Barker, E. T., Seltzer, M. M., Floyd, F., Greenberg, J., Orsmond, G., & Bolt, D. (2010). The relative risk and timing of divorce in families of children with an autism spectrum disorder. *Journal of Family Psychology, 24*(4), 449.

Fernell, E., Eriksson, M. A., & Gillberg, C. (2013). Early diagnosis of autism and impact on prognosis: A narrative review. *Clinical Epidemiology*, 33–43.

Freedman, B. H., Kalb, L. G., Zablotsky, B., & Stuart, E. A. (2012). Relationship status among parents of children with autism spectrum disorders: A population-based study. *Journal of Autism and Developmental Disorders, 42*(4), 539–548.

Howlin, P., & Asgharian, A. (1999). The diagnosis of autism and Asperger syndrome: findings from a survey of 770 families. *Developmental Medicine and Child Neurology, 41*(12), 834–839.

Moore, V., & Goodson, S. (2003). How well does early diagnosis of autism stand the test of time? Follow-up study of children assessed for autism at age 2 and development of an early diagnostic service. *Autism, 7*(1), 47–63.

Naseef, R., & Freedman, B. (2012). A diagnosis of autism is not a prognosis of divorce. *Autism Advocate, 8*, 12.

Rondeau, E., Klein, L. S., Masse, A., Bodeau, N., Cohen, D., & Guilé, J. M. (2011). Is pervasive developmental disorder not otherwise specified less stable than autistic disorder? A meta-analysis. *Journal of Autism and Developmental Disorders, 41*, 1267–1276.

Seltzer, M. M., Krauss, M. W., Orsmond, G. I., & Vestal, C. (2000). Families of adolescents and adults with autism: Uncharted territory. In *International review of research in mental retardation* (Vol. 23, pp. 267–294). Academic Press.

Woodgate, R. L., Ateah, C., & Secco, L. (2008). Living in a world of our own: The experience of parents who have a child with autism. *Qualitative Health Research, 18*(8), 1075–1083. doi:10.1177/1049732308320112

Zirkel, P. A. (2011). Autism litigation under the IDEA: A new meaning of "disproportionality"? *Special Education Leadership, 24*, 92–103.

5 Debunking the IEP

Empowering Families through Knowledge

Gwendolyn Edwards

Clinical Case: Brendan, 7

In understanding the assessment and Individualized Education Program (IEP) processes, it is helpful to apply the information to a real-life scenario. Therefore, let us look at the assessment and IEP process for Brendan and what his family went through to help obtain the diagnosis and accommodations he needed to have a more successful academic and emotional experience at school.

Brendan Thomas is a white male who is seven years old and is starting the second grade. At the first parent-teacher conference meeting in the fall, Mr. and Mrs. Thomas were approached by Brendan's second grade teacher, Ms. Heather, to talk about some of the behaviors she had noticed in the classroom and to inquire whether they had seen some of these in their home. During the discussion, Ms. Heather mentioned that Brendan seemed to have a hard time focusing and shifting tasks, a preference for following routine, repetitive behaviors, difficulty with social cues, strains with social relationships, emotional outbursts, trouble with social interactions, and noise sensitivity. Brendan's parents were a little surprised since she was the first teacher to bring this to their attention; however, they had noticed that Brendan had been struggling at school because he said that he did not have any friends and did not like his classroom this year. Ms. Heather asked if there was any concern about Brendan's behavior before and said that he may benefit from an evaluation to determine whether he meets the criteria for accommodations, which could greatly improve his overall experience. Mr. and Mrs. Thomas felt shocked, upset, anxious, and guilty when the IEP was suggested. They anxiously asked many questions, like "What is an evaluation? Is that connected to an IEP? What's the difference between an IEP and a 504? Is this necessary? Is this going to make him stand out?" Once the initial wave of emotions decreased, Mr. and Mrs. Thomas discussed some of the behaviors that Ms. Heather reported in the classroom, and they reflected on their experiences at home; they recognized

DOI: 10.4324/9781003451266-5

that Brendan was also displaying those behaviors Ms. Heather described. Upon further discussion, Mr. and Mrs. Thomas realized that they had always adjusted to Brendan to make things easier at home for him and for them as a family, and maybe that if he had some of the accommodations at school that they had already implemented in the home, he would enjoy school more. Mrs. Thomas remembered that her friend Jane went through this evaluation process a couple of years ago with her daughter Jenna. Mrs. Thomas reached out to Jane to ask about this evaluation process and how they got the process started with the school. Jane sent over an example of the letter she submitted to request an evaluation and suggested that Mrs. Thomas do the same for Brendan. A couple of days later, Mrs. Thomas wrote up an official request for an IEP evaluation and submitted it to the school.

While looking at all aspects of an IEP, Brendan's case will be discussed throughout this chapter to apply the steps of this process to a case example. In looking at starting this process, the first step to getting an IEP for a child is to request a special education eligibility evaluation from the special education administrator at the school. While the school district might also request an evaluation first, written consent is required to begin the evaluation either way. However, the most important aspect of this first step is to submit a written request. Once that happens, the initial evaluation must be completed within 60 days of the school receiving consent from the caregiver. Additionally, it is important to know that the school must share the detailed evaluation plan; therefore, everyone is aware of the testing and observation the child will undergo. Assessments will be discussed later in this chapter. The assessment section will be helpful for parents and caregivers to become familiar with tests that school districts use during the evaluation and are the most appropriate tests to provide a basis for developing an IEP for the child. Additionally, the following rights and tips may be helpful: One may have the right to suggest changes to the evaluation plan. For example, if one feels there are potential areas for evaluation that may not have been included, one may request to meet with the assigned evaluator before the evaluation begins, which can give one an opportunity to ask questions about the tests to be performed and the other evaluation methods to be utilized.

What goes into a Psychological Assessment?

During the evaluation process, one can expect objective tests to evaluate the child in areas such as general intelligence, reading comprehension, psychological states, social development, and physical abilities. It is also helpful for the caregivers to provide as much detail and background information regarding their child's developmental, physical, and social milestones as possible. What are milestones? Developmental milestones are a set of goals or markers that a child is expected to achieve during maturation. They are categorized into five domains: gross motor, fine motor, language, cognitive, and social-emotional and behavioral. Recently, the Centers for Disease Control and Prevention (CDC) has updated the criteria for developmental milestones, specifically what would be defined as a delay (Centers for Disease Control and Prevention, 2023a). Developmental milestone information is readily available on the Internet (just be mindful of the source that is used). Any pediatrician's office will have information regarding the child's developmental milestones at every age. Within a psychological interview, it is not unusual for the questions to revolve around milestones, behaviors growing up and in the home, sleeping habits, eating habits, family history of mental health, child's history of mental health, anything medical or physical going on for the child or in the family, and any major stressors going on in the family at that time, to gather all information about the child for the evaluation. Additionally, comprehensive information such as teacher and parent reports, evaluations by experts specializing in the child's disability, letters from the child's pediatrician or counselor, and evidence of school performance will be considered in the evaluation. At the end, there will be a conclusion regarding the child's eligibility for special education and recommendations for meeting the child's specific needs.

In Brendan's case, Mr. and Mrs. Thomas met with the school's evaluator, the school district's psychologist, to provide a clinical interview and discuss different observations they had noticed over the years. Mrs. Thomas stated that she did not experience any complications with her pregnancy with Brendan, and he was born on time. At the time of Brendan's birth, Mrs. Thomas was 35 years old, and Mr. Thomas was 38 years old. As a child, Brendan was described as difficult to soothe and very colicky as a baby. He was also difficult to entertain as he would seemingly get bored with things easily and was unable to entertain or occupy himself. Mrs. Thomas stated that Brendan was often observed looking around but not making eye contact or smiling at anyone during infancy. She was worried about his eyesight and had Brendan's eyesight evaluated multiple times but was always told there was no concern. At first, the parents reported no concerns in regard to Brendan's eating. However, over the past couple years Brendan has been more extreme regarding his preferences on what he would or would not like to eat, and more so stating that the temperature and texture of his food bother him greatly. For example, Brendan will not eat food while it is warm; he has to wait for it to get cold before he can eat it. Mr. and Mrs. Thomas reported that as he has grown up,

Brendan has met all milestones early or within normal limits, and his hearing and vision were reported to be acceptable. Currently, Brendan wears glasses due to having difficulty seeing at a distance. In discussing what they have observed socially for Brendan, Mr. and Mrs. Thomas commented that Brendan's social skills and peer relations were always difficult. They stated that Brendan did not have friends when he was growing up but recently had made two or three close friends. Brendan was reported to play better with peers who share interests similar to his, such as dinosaurs, classical music, and a game he likes to play, which is Roblox. In the home, Mrs. Thomas stated that Brendan prefers a routine and likes to know what to expect throughout the day, especially in the morning, which has caused some disagreements between him and his parents. Mrs. Thomas stated that she also noticed Brendan's noise sensitivity, which she felt began at a young age when Brendan would be upset and difficult to console when presented with loud noises, such as in a movie theater or at fireworks. Brendan also presents with social and emotional behavioral concerns that Mr. and Mrs. Thomas reported in the home, such as difficulty transitioning from one task to the next, rocking when nervous, doing repetitive behaviors, hitting himself in the head when angry, and sometimes needing reminders not to engage in socially immature behaviors, such as being unable to dress himself, becoming impatient easily, and seeming unaware of his surroundings. At times, Mrs. Thomas stated that she has had to repeat directions multiple times before Brendan completes the objective, which has caused her to create chore charts and rewards systems, which have had some success in helping to remind Brendan of what he needs to do when asked. Additionally, there are concerns about Brendan's ability to care for himself in a developmentally appropriate way. Mrs. Thomas stated that she has to help him daily with dressing and grooming due to his difficulties in maintaining attention and focus to autonomously complete the task, along with difficulties with sensory aspects of washing himself, brushing his hair and teeth, and getting dressed. Mrs. Thomas said multiple times that if she doesn't help him get ready in the morning, Brendan will not engage in these activities and would not see anything wrong with it.

Assessment Tools that are Commonly Used for an Autism Assessment

Below are commonly used assessments, but this list is not exhaustive, as there are always new and updated versions of different psychological assessments. The assessments listed below and the domains described are commonly used assessments within the school setting as well as for assessing for autism.

Cognitive Functioning

Cognitive or intellectual functioning testing is recommended as part of a comprehensive autism spectrum disorder (ASD) evaluation (Johnson & Myers, 2007; Daily, 2016). Cognitive testing typically encompasses measures that assess the strengths and weaknesses in both verbal and nonverbal abilities, problem-solving, concept formation, reasoning, style of learning, memory skills, and other domains. Measures that are most widely used for assessing cognitive functioning are:

• Wechsler Preschool and Primary Scale of Intelligence, Third Edition (WIPPSI-IV; Wechsler, 2012)
• Wechsler Intelligence Scale for Children, Fifth Edition (WISC-V; Weschler, 2014)
• Woodcock-Johnson III Test of Cognitive Abilities (WJ-III; Woodcock, McGrew & Mather 2001, 2007a)
• Stanford-Binet Intelligence Scales, Fifth Edition (SB5; Roid, 2003)

Adaptive Functioning

Assessment in adaptive behavior is also recommended for any individual with a possible ASD. Adaptive functioning includes how an individual can function within conceptual, social, and practical domains (Daily, 2016). Scales and assessments that measure adaptive functioning are the following:

• Vineland Adaptive Behavioral Scales, Second Edition (Sparrow et al., 2005)
• Adaptive Behavior Assessment System, Second Edition (ABAS-II; Harrison & Oakland, 2003)

Autism Scales

There are several scales, including rating scales, interviews, and observational assessments, that measure specific symptoms related to ASD. The most commonly used are:

• Childhood Autism Rating Scale, Second Edition (CARS2; Schopler, Reichler, DeVellis, Daly, 1980)
• Gilliam Autism Rating Scale, Third Edition (GARS-3; Gilliam, 2013)

The Autism Diagnostic Interview-Revised (ADI-R; Lord et al., 1994) is a semistructured interview with the parent or caregiver that requires extensive training to administer and, therefore, is often used primarily for research (Daily, 2016). Currently, one of the most widely used assessment measures is the Autism Diagnostic Observation Schedule, Second Edition (ADOS-2; Lord et al., 2012). This standardized observational assessment measures social effects, communication, reciprocal social interactions, and restricted and repetitive behaviors.

Academic Functioning

Achievement measures may be given to evaluate an individual's academic functioning. The most common achievement tests given to an individual with ASD are:

- Woodcock-Johnson IV Tests of Achievement (Woodcock et al., 2001; Schrank et al., 2014)
- Wechsler Individual Achievement Test, Third Edition (Wechsler, 2009)

Emotional and Behavioral Functioning

Comprehensive evaluations for ASD also include social, emotional, and behavioral rating scales. One of the most used general measures, which includes teacher, parent, and self-report forms, is the Behavior Assessment System for Children-2 (BASC-2; Reynolds & Kamphau, 2004). The BASC-2 evaluation looks at symptoms related to depression, anxiety, attention deficit hyperactivity disorder (ADHD), behavior disorders, psychosis, and tic disorders, as well as clinical information specific to ASD. Similarly, the Achenbach System of Empirically Based Assessment (ASEBA), and specifically the Child Behavior Checklist (CBCL: Achenbach & Rescorla, 2001) are parent-report measures that assess symptoms of depression, anxiety, somatic complaints, obsessive-compulsive behaviors, attention problems, social difficulties, aggressive behaviors, and atypical behaviors within the child, and the CBCL version for children ages three months to five years also provides information related to ASD. Given the comorbidity that occurs in ASD and ADHD, it's important to also evaluate for ADHD symptoms. A common rating scale may include the Conners' Rating Scale, third edition (Conners, 2008), which assesses symptoms of ADHD, defiant disorder, and conduct disorder (Daily, 2016).

Language Functioning

Given the many social pragmatic language and communication difficulties individuals with ASD possess, it is also important to have a speech-language evaluation. A speech-language pathologist can assess language skills, social competency, phonology, dyspraxia, apraxia, articulation, hearing, voice tone and volume, oral motor skills, and verbal fluency (Daily, 2016).

Social Communication

For pragmatic language, it is important to use some observational data taken during a conversation with the individual that evaluates the function of communication, the organization of turns and topics and conversation, flexible use of language forms and relationships specific context, the use of presupposition, and conversational manners.

Sensory Functioning

One of the most frequently used assessment measures for sensory functioning is the Sensory Profile (Dunn, 1999), which is an apparent questionnaire. Clinical observations, as well as the Sensory Integration and Praxis Test, can be helpful in assessing sensory function (Ayers, 1989).

Motor Functioning

There are several assessment measures that assess fine and gross motor skills. Some of the fine motor measures include:

- Beery-Buktenica Developmental Test of Visual-Motor Integration, Fifth Edition (Beery& Beery, 2006)
- Bender Visual Motor Gestalt Test (Bender-Gestalt II; Brannigan & Decker, 2003)
- The Peabody Developmental Motor Scales, Second Edition (PDMS-2; Folio & Fewell, 2000)

To assess only gross motor skills, these assessments may be used:

- Tests of Gross Motor Development, Second Edition (Ulrich, 2000)
- Clinical Observation of Motor and Postural Skills (COMPS), Second Edition (Wilson et al., 1994, 2000)
- Movement Assessment Battery for Children, Second Edition (Henderson et al., 2007)

In Brendan's case, he was administered the Weschler Intelligence Scale for Children, fifth edition (WISC-V), and the Autism Diagnostic Observation Schedule, second edition (ADOS-2) by the school psychologist. Additionally, Brendan's parents and teachers were asked to fill out multiple rating scales, such as the Autism Spectrum Rating Scale (ASRS), Behavioral Rating Inventory of Executive Function, second edition (BRIEF-2); Conner's 3; and the Social Responsiveness Scales, second edition (SRS-2). It is important to note that this is an example of a psychological assessment battery (group of assessments), and that while some of these assessments will be standard, especially in assessments for autism such as the ADOS, it will be at the discretion of the psychologist to select the assessments that are most appropriate for the question being asked at that time. For Brendan, the main question that was being asked was why he was displaying behaviors in the classroom such as having a hard time focusing, shifting tasks, showing a preference for following routine, engaging in repetitive behaviors, having difficulty with social cues, experiencing difficulties with social relationships, having emotional outbursts, trouble with social interactions, and experiencing noise sensitivity. The assessments that were selected for Brendan will help provide guidance and direction for the next steps for helping Brendan in the classroom and can provide some insight into services that his parents could investigate to help him more at home. Some school districts have access to occupational therapists and speech therapists as well, and these two, among other disciplines, may provide other assessments that would be included in the school setting if it would be appropriate for the individual. In Brendan's assessment, it was found that he presented with symptoms that fit the criteria of both ASD, Level 2, and ADHD, Combined Presentation. Once the report was given to Mr. and Mrs. Thomas, it was determined that Brendan qualified for an IEP, and a meeting was set up within 30 days of the assessment being completed.

The Evaluation is Completed ... Now What?

The psychological evaluation is complete and should provide guidance as to why behaviors are happening in the classroom. In most cases, it should provide a diagnosis for the child and direction as to what needs to happen next to best benefit the child. After the assessment is completed and provided to the caregivers, there is a meeting to review the evaluation and recommendations and help decide what special education and related services the student needs. The next two sections will discuss in depth what that process looks like, especially with an IEP team, an IEP meeting, the writing of the IEP, and what happens after the IEP is implemented. All the information gathered within the evaluation process and reports from the child's teachers will help describe the student's present levels of educational performance. Knowing how the student is currently performing in school will help to develop the IEP as well as develop annual goals to address those areas where the student has an identified educational need.

What if the family disagrees with the school's evaluation outcome? If the school's evaluation concludes that the child is not eligible for an IEP, as a caregiver, one has the right to an Independent Education Evaluation (IEE) at the school district's expense. As in previous requests, it is important to also make this request in writing. The school district must cover the cost of the IEE or else file a due process complaint to request a hearing to show that its evaluation is appropriate. The school district is required to consider the results of the independent evaluation when determining eligibility for a child (Office of Special Education and Rehabilitative Services, 2000 and 2006; The National Autism Association, 2018).

Who should be a Part of the IEP Team?

Certain individuals must be involved in writing a child's IEP by law. The school district will assign a case manager or team leader to oversee the child's IEP and progress, most likely a special education teacher. The team will also include a general education teacher (if the child spends any part of their day in a general education classroom), a school administrator (such as the principal), and a school psychologist or social worker to review assessments and so forth. The team can also include other teachers, such as a music teacher or a reading specialist, as well as professionals providing related services, including a speech pathologist, physical therapist, or behavioral aide. As previously discussed in other chapters, there are different times for advocacy in an individual's life, and if there are other people in the child's life who may be helpful in providing information or recommendations throughout the IEP process, like a doctor or even a close friend, including them in this process as well, would be helpful. Some individuals might decide to bring an advocate or an attorney to a meeting, especially if a disagreement or a dispute needs to be resolved. These people must work together as a team to write the child's IEP. Additionally, it is important to note that the meeting to write the IEP must be held within 30 calendar days of deciding that the child is eligible for special education and related services. Each of these team members brings important information to the IEP meeting to help assist the child by sharing information and working together to add to the team's understanding of the child and what services the child needs.

Parents and caregivers are key members of the IEP team. They know the child very well and can talk about the child's strengths and needs as well as their ideas for enhancing their child's education. Caregivers can offer insight into how the child learns, what their interests are, and other aspects of the child that would be beneficial for the school to know. The IEP meeting can generate a discussion so that team members can talk about what the child needs to work on at school, and caregivers can report on whether the skills the child is learning at school are being used at home. In preparing for an IEP meeting, it can be helpful for individuals to write out a list of programs, services, and goals that benefit the child and that they would like to be incorporated into the IEP plan if possible. Being as clear as possible with goals, wishes, and expectations, as well as being respectful and understanding of the opinions and findings of the school professionals, can lead to a more fulfilling IEP meeting experience, which will ultimately benefit the child.

Other important members of the IEP team will include teachers that the child engages with on a regular basis. At least one of the child's regular education teachers must be on the IEP team if the child is (or maybe) participating in the regular education environment. The regular educa- tion teacher has a great deal to share with the team. The child's teacher can provide direct behavioral observations that they have noticed in the classroom. Teachers can also discuss support that is going to be needed in the classroom for the child to advance toward annual goals, to progress within the general curriculum, to participate in activities, and to educate their peers.

If the child is already engaged in working with special education teachers, their contributions to the IEP team would also be important information. Because special education teachers have a different specialized training background from general teachers, they can provide suggestions around how to modify the general curriculum to help the child learn, the supple- mentary aids and services that the child may need to be successful in the regular classroom, how to modify testing, and other aspects of individual- izing instruction to meet the student's unique needs.

The individual representing the school system is also a valuable team member; as they have this role, they know a great deal about special edu- cation services and educating children with disabilities. The school rep- resentative can talk about the necessary school resources. It is important that this individual has the authority to commit resources and be able to ensure that whatever services are set out in the IEP will be provided. In some school districts, a parent advocate could also be a part of the IEP team on behalf of the caregivers and child. The advocate can be extremely helpful with navigating the IEP and knowing how to advocate for services for the child, and helping the caregivers navigate the ins and outs of an IEP, especially if it is their first time. All this information throughout the IEP process can be overwhelming, and having an additional individual to help advocate for the child's needs can be such a relief for caregivers.

The IEP team may also include additional individuals with knowledge or special expertise about the child. The caregivers or the school system can invite these individuals to participate on the team. For example, caregivers may invite an advocate who knows the child, such as a professional with special expertise about the child and their disability, or others (such as a vocational educator who has been working with the child) who can talk about the child's strengths and/or needs. Depending on the child's individual needs, some related service professionals attending the IEP meeting or otherwise helping to develop the IEP might include occupational or physical therapists, adaptive physical education providers, psychologists, or speech-language pathologists. Last but not least, the student may also be a member of the IEP team if this is appropriate. If transition service needs or transition services are going to be discussed at the meeting, the student must be invited to attend. More and more students are participating in and even leading their own IEP meetings. This allows them to have a strong voice in their education and can teach them much about self-advocacy and self-determination.

Once an IEP team is established, they will meet to discuss specific information about the child. This information will include the child's strengths, the parents' ideas for enhancing their child's education, the results of recent evaluations or reevaluations, and information on how the child has done on state and district-wide tests. In addition, the IEP team must consider other factors, such as how to help the child advance toward the annual goals, how to be involved in and progress in the general curriculum, how to participate in extracurricular and nonacademic activities, and how to be educated with and participate with other children with disabilities and nondisabled children.

The Initial Meeting and Writing the IEP

Once the team is established, they will then meet to write the child's IEP. The IEP will include the services and support the school will provide for the child. If the IEP team decides that a child needs a particular device or service (including an intervention, accommodation, or other program modification), the team must write this information in the IEP. For example, consider a child whose behavior interferes with learning. The team would consider positive and effective ways to address that behavior. The team would discuss the positive behavioral interventions, strategies, and supports the child needs to learn, to control or manage their behavior.

An IEP form starts with the student's current level of performance at school. The performance review will cover academic performance, such as test results and grades, but also go well beyond that to include behavioral challenges, social skills, communication abilities, learning styles, and sensory or motor skill development. All this information will come from assessments and observations by team members. Clearly defining the child's current strengths and challenges will help build the foundation of a successful education plan that will allow the child to thrive to the best of their abilities inside and outside the classroom. Together, the IEP team will define goals for the child. It is critical that the goals for the IEP be meaningful and measurable. These goals essentially drive the education process for the child. Therefore, if the goals are not meaningful, all the resources and support the team is putting in place to accomplish them will not be effectively used. Additionally, if the goals are not measurable, it will be difficult to monitor how the child is doing in school. Each of the goals must include information about how and when progress toward that specific goal will be measured. The IEP should make it very clear how team members can monitor how well the child is doing in each goal. As the goals are clearly defined, the IEP will also define all the supports and services the child will receive at school in order to reach the stated goals, for example, recommended special education programs and related services like speech therapy or psychological counseling, as well as the specific accommodations or modifications that will be made to support the education plan, such as testing modifications, special seating, or inter-preter services. Last, the IEP will include information about these extra resources' frequency, duration, location, and start date so that the team is aware of where, when, and how these services are provided.

When the IEP is completed, the caregiver must be provided a copy of the plan at no cost. This is explicitly stated in the IDEA (please refer back to Chapter 4 regarding the discussion of the IDEA), and everyone who will be involved in implementing the IEP must have access to the document. Individuals needing access to this document would be regular education teachers, special education teachers, speech or occupational therapists, and any other service provider responsible for the child's education. Providing these individuals with a copy of this document assists each of these indi-viduals in knowing what their specific responsibilities are for carrying out the child's IEP. It is important to note that before the school can provide a child with special education and related services for the first time, the child's parents must give their written permission.

In addition, the child's placement, defining exactly where the IEP will be carried out, must be decided. The IEP team serves as the group making the placement decision; however, it is important to note that caregivers have the right to be members of the group that decides the educational placement of the child. According to the IDEA's Least Restrictive Environment (LRE) requirements, placement decisions must be made. These requirements state that, to the maximum extent appropriate, children with disabilities must be educated with children who do not have disabilities. The law also clearly states that special classes, separate schools, or removal of children with disabilities from the regular educational environment may occur only if the nature or severity of the child's disability is such that services cannot be achieved satisfactorily (Office of Special Education and

Rehabilitative Services, 2000; The National Autism Association, 2018). A school system may meet its obligation to ensure that the child has an appropriate placement available by providing an appropriate program for the child on its own, contracting with another agency to provide an appropriate program, or utilizing some other mechanism or arrangement that is consistent with the IDEA for providing or paying for an appropriate program for the child. The placement will be based on the IEP and the appropriate placement option for the child. For example, can the child be educated in the regular classroom, with proper aids and supports? If the child cannot be educated in the regular classroom, even with appropriate aids and supports, then the placement group will talk about other placements for the child.

What power does the caregiver have to modify the IEP? Can a child's IEP be revised to accommodate a caregiver's request? Absolutely. After the initial IEP meeting, the caregivers and the school will sign the plan that was developed. If there are lingering questions or areas that are not fully answered or do not feel resolved, the caregivers should not sign the IEP until they feel comfortable and confident in the plan. It is important to monitor progress closely so that the team can address issues as soon as they arise and update the plan accordingly.

Transition Services

When the child reaches high school, it is important that the IEP team work out a comprehensive plan for their transition to adulthood. These transition services are implemented to support the individual plan and should begin in the early to mid-teen years so the student is as prepared as possible for life after the traditional K-12 education ends. Similar to the IEP, the transition plan should be unique to the student's individual strengths, challenges, needs, and wants for his future. Resources and services that are available to older teens/young adults are fully explained in chapters 8 and 9 of this book.

Implementing, Revising, and Reviewing the IEP

Once the IEP is written, the student will be provided with special education and related services as listed in the IEP. These services include all supplementary aids and services and program modifications that the IEP team, including the caregiver, has identified as necessary for the student to advance appropriately toward his or her IEP goals. As previously discussed, it is important for every individual involved in providing services to the student to know and understand their responsibilities for carrying out the IEP. Teamwork is a huge aspect of making the child's IEP successful. Taking a team approach allows the integration of multiple disciplines of professionals to benefit the student. Providing a space to share expertise and insights can improve student results. Another key aspect of success with the IEP is communication between the home and school. Caregivers can share information about what is happening at home and build upon what the child is learning at school. If the child is having difficulty at school, caregivers may be able to offer insight to the school and explore possible reasons and solutions. The law requires regular progress reports to help parents and schools monitor the child's progress toward his or her annual goals (Office of Special Education and Rehabilitative Services, 2000; The National Autism Association, 2018). It is important to know if the child is not making the expected progress, or if he or she has progressed much faster than expected. Parents and school personnel can address the child's needs as those needs become evident.

To monitor the goals and progress of the child and the IEP, the team must review the child's IEP at least once a year. During the annual meeting, the team will discuss the child's progress or deficiency of expected progress toward the annual goals and curriculum. For example, if the child was reevaluated and new observations or information was found from this reevaluation, or there was new updated information from the child's caregivers, it would be helpful to discuss all of this at the meeting. While the IDEA requires this IEP review at least once a year, the team may review and revise the IEP more often. Either the parents or the school can ask to hold an IEP meeting to revise the child's IEP. For example, the child may not be making progress toward his or her IEP goals, and his or her teacher or parents may become concerned. On the other hand, the child may have met most or all of the goals in the IEP, and new ones need to be written. In either case, the IEP team would meet to revise the IEP.

While there may be some variation in IEP forms from state to state, most will include: an explanation of the extent to which the child will be removed from his peers (to ensure the child is in the Least Restrictive Environment (LRE) as mandated by IDEA); an explanation of a child's exemption from statewide assessments and a list of alternative assessments that will be used, if applicable; specific sections about supports related to transportation needs, assistive technology requirements, extended school year services eligibility, and so on (Office of Special Education and Rehabilitative Services, 2000; The National Autism Association, 2018).

Disputing an IEP

If a caregiver is not happy with the IEP or how the IEP is being implemented at the school, they can dispute the IEP and request an informal meeting to resolve any disagreement with the school. Being able to reach out to the

IEP team or meet directly with the teachers responsible for the implementation of the IEP to share any concerns can be crucial. The IEP process can be emotional and overwhelming at times. To help process some of these feelings and emotions that can arise, it can help to present and write out any thoughts and questions prior to the meeting. However, if an informal conversation or a planned IEP meeting does not resolve the issue, there are several steps one can take by law under the IDEA. First, start by writing a letter to the school that outlines concerns and proposes solutions. The next step is often to request a formal mediation session or a conversation between the school and a neutral third party present who has expertise in special education and IEP matters. The goal is for the mediator to help the two parties explore compromises and reach a solution that is agreeable to everyone. The mediator does not make the decision, but rather facilitates a constructive conversation that hopefully results in an agreement. A mediation session is much less formal and confrontational than a hearing. If a solution can be met, then that solution will be documented in writing and be binding between both parties.

Due Process Hearing

If an agreement cannot be reached through an informal meeting or mediator meeting, then the next step is a due process hearing. There is a difference between disagreeing with the child's IEP or with the services being provided to the child, and finding that the school is not fulfilling its legal obligations required by law under the IDEA to provide a "free appropriate public education" in the LRE. Mediations and due process hearings focus on issues regarding the education that the child is getting at school; filing a state complaint is essentially formally accusing the school district of violating the law (Office of Special Education and Rehabilitative Services, 2000 and 2006; The National Autism Association, 2018).

To start the due process hearing, a complaint must be filed with the school district, and a copy must be sent to the state department of education responsible for special education. Under the IDEA, the complaint must be filed within two years of when the issue began or the violation occurred. A due process complaint must contain the name of the child, the address of the residence of the child, the name of the school the child is attending, a description of the nature of the problem, including relevant facts, and a proposed resolution of the problem to the extent known and available to the party at the time (Office of Special Education and Rehabilitative Services, 2000, 2006; The National Autism Association, 2018). Upon filing a complaint, the applicable government agency will investigate the complaint, which will usually entail meeting with the individual who submitted the complaint and providing an opportunity to present additional information, review the evidence and records, and then decide. The IDEA requires a decision to be issued within 60 days of filing the complaint.

In this situation, it can be common for caregivers to hire an attorney to prepare for and assist them with a hearing. Hiring an advocate or an attorney to help is sometimes necessary to bridge the gap and ensure that the child's rights are not being violated and that their needs are being met at school. A hearing is a formal process that involves the child, caregivers, and the school district making opening and closing statements and presenting written evidence and witness testimony. A neutral third party, a hearing officer, will preside over the hearing and will make a final, binding, written determination regarding the dispute. Either party has the right to appeal the written determination to a state or federal court. Each state handles these complaints differently, so be sure to research the process in your state thoroughly before moving forward.

Conclusion

In conclusion, navigating the IEP process for children with autism within a school setting is a multifaceted journey that demands unwavering dedication, collaboration, and empathy from all involved stakeholders. Throughout this chapter, we have explored the intricacies of this process, aiming to equip parents, educators, and professionals with the knowledge and tools necessary to advocate effectively for the educational needs of children with autism. Understanding the IEP process begins with recognizing the unique strengths, challenges, and individualized needs of each child. Comprehensive assessments conducted by a multidisciplinary team provide the foundation for developing meaningful and measurable goals that address academic, social, and behavioral objectives. By prioritizing a child-centered approach, we ensure that the IEP reflects not only academic benchmarks but also the holistic development and well-being of the student. Effective communication lies at the heart of successful IEP implementation. Parents, educators, therapists, and other specialists must collaborate closely, sharing insights, observations, and feedback to inform decision-making and goal-setting. Building strong partnerships based on trust, respect, and open dialogue fosters a supportive environment in which the child's best interests remain paramount. As we navigate the IEP process, it is essential to remain flexible and responsive to the evolving needs of the child. Regular progress monitoring and ongoing evaluation enable us to gauge the effectiveness of interventions and make necessary adjustments to ensure continued growth and success. By embracing a dynamic and iterative approach, we can adapt strategies and supports to meet the changing needs of the child over time. Central to the IEP process is the provision of appropriate accommodations and modifications that facilitate access to the curriculum and promote meaningful participation in the learning environment. By tailoring support to the individual preferences and learning styles of each child, we empower them to reach their full potential.

Transition planning represents a pivotal aspect of the IEP process, preparing children with autism for successful transitions between grade levels, educational settings, and life stages. Whether transitioning from early intervention to preschool, from elementary to middle school, or from high school to postsecondary education and adulthood, careful planning and collaboration ensure continuity of support and a seamless transition process.

The IEP process serves as a vehicle for empowerment, advocacy, and inclusion. By actively involving children with autism in the planning and decision-making process, we promote self-determination and autonomy, fostering a sense of ownership over their educational journey. Additionally, advocating for inclusive practices and environments within the school community ensures that children with autism are valued, respected, and fully included in all aspects of school life. By working together, we empower children with autism to thrive academically, socially, and emotionally, ensuring that they receive the individualized support and opportunities they need to reach their full potential and laying the foundation for a more inclusive and equitable future.

References

Achenbach, T. M., & Rescorla, L. (2001). *ASEBA school-age forms & profiles.* Burlington: Aseba.

Ayres, A. J. (1989). Sensory integration and praxis test (SIPT). *Los Angeles: Western Psychological Services.*

Beery, K. E. & Beery, N.A. (2006). *The Beery-Buktenica developmental test of visual-motor integration with supplemental developmental tests of visual perception and motor coordination for children and adults and stepping stones age norms from birth to age six: Administration, scoring and teaching manual,* 5th ed. Minneapolis, MN, USA: NCS Pearson, Inc.

Brannigan. G., & Decker, S. (2003). *Bender visual -moto Gestalt test,(Bender Gestalt II).* Itasca, IL: Riverside Publishing.

Center for Disease Control and Prevention. (2023a, June 6). *CDC's developmental milestones.* Centers for Disease Control and Prevention. www.cdc.gov/ncbddd/actearly/milestones/index.html

Conners, C. K. (2008). Conners' rating scale-revised: Manual. Tonawanda, NY: Multi-Health Systems.

Daily, M. C. (2016). *The key to autism: An evidence-based workbook for assessing and treating children & adolescents: Practical strategies for organization,* social communication, self-regulation, and solving challenging behaviors. Pesi Publishing & Media.

Dunn, W. (1999). *Short sensory profile*. San Antonio, TX: Psychological Corporation.

Folio, M. R., & Fewell, R. R. (2000). *Peabody Developmental Motor Scales– Second Edition (PDMS-2)*. PRO-ED.

Gilliam, J. E. (2013). *Gilliam Autism Rating Scale- Third Edition*. Austin, TX: Pro-Ed.

Harrison, P. L., & Oakland, T. (2003). *Adaptive Behavior Assessment System– Second Edition (ABAS-II)*. The Psychological Corporation.

Johnson, C. P., & Myers, S. M. (2007). Identification and evaluation of children with autism spectrum disorders. *Pediatrics*, 120(5), 1183–1215.

Lord, C., Luyster, R., Gotham, K., & Gutherie, W. J. (2012). Autism diagnostic observation schedule-Toddler module. *Los Angeles: Western Psychological Services*.

Lord, C., Rutter, M., & Le Couteur, A. (1994). Autism Diagnostic Interview Revised: a revised version of a diagnostic interview for caregivers of individuals with possible pervasive development disorders. *Journal of Autism and Developmental Disorders*, 24(5), 659–685.

Office of Special Education and Rehabilitative Services, Heumann, J., Warlick, K., Richards, C., Price-Ellingstad, D., Reynolds, J., Ringer, L., Ryder, R., & Sheridan, S. (2000). *1 A guide to the individualized education program*. Washington, DC: Office of Special Education and Rehabilitative Services, U.S. Department of Education.

Office of Special Education and Rehabilitative Services, Department of Education. (2006, August 14). Title 34. *34 CFR Part 300 Subpart D – Individualized Education Programs*. www.ecfr.gov/current/title-34/subtitle-B/chapter-III/part-300/subpart-D/subject-group-ECFR28b07e67452ed7a/

Reynolds, C. R., & Kamphaus, R. W. (2004). *BASC-2: Behavior assessment system for children*. John Wiley & Son, Inc.

Roid, G. H. (2003). *Stanford-Binet Intelligence Scales, Fifth Edition*. Itasca, IL: Riverside.

Schrank, F., Mather, N., & McGrew, K. (2014). *Woodcock-Johnson IV Tests of Achievement*. Rolling Meadows, IL: Riverside.

Sparrow, S. S., Cicchetti, D. V., & Balla, D. A. (2005). *Vineland Adaptive Behavioral Scales, Second Edition*. Circle Pine: MN: American Guidance Service.

The National Autism Association. (2018). *ASD & the IEP process*. ASD & the IEP Process A Resource Provided by the National Autism Association Tips & Tools for an Effective Individualized Education Plan (IEP). https://nationalautismassociation.org/wp-content/uploads/2018/08/NAA-IEP-Toolkit.pdf

Ulrich, D. (2000). *Test of Gross Motor Development- Second Edition* (TGMD-2). Austin, TX: ProEd, Inc.

Wechsler, D. (2009) *Wechsler Individual Achievement Test(3rd ed.)*. San Antonio, TX: PCS Pearson.

Wechsler, D. (2012) *Wechsler Preschool and Primary Scale of Intelligence- Fourth Edition*. San Antonio, TX: PCS Pearson.

Wechsler, D. (2014) *Wechsler Intelligence Scale for Children- Fifth Edition.* San Antonio, TX: PCS Pearson.

Wilson, B., Pollack, N., Kaplan, B., & Law, M. (2000) Clinical Observation of Moto and Postural Skills: Administration and scoring manual, Second edition. Framingham, MA: Therapro, Inc.

Woodcock, R. W., McGrew, K. S.& Mather, N. (2001, 2007a). *Woodcock Johnson III Tests of Achievement.* Rolling Meadows, IL: Riverside.

6   Subsystems

Clinical Challenges of Subsystems with a Focus on Siblings

Britney Fontes

How Family Members Impact One Another

Each family member does not live in a bubble but instead exists in a multi-faceted, complex, and unique system that is multidirectional and influenced by various factors. In other words, what might appear to be an individual problem will likely affect multiple family members. Let us take a step away from autism and use an example that many families might experience. It is not uncommon that, at some point, a parent gets a new job. This new job might seem like an individual experience; however, a shift in one person's life most often affects the people around them. For example, a new job might mean the entire family has to relocate and move to a new neighborhood, school, or even state. A new job might impose financial burdens or access to more resources. A new job could require parents to work a new shift with additional hours, which may affect how and when the family can partake in activities such as meals, bedtime, or daily chores. When a family has to shift their schedule, location, or daily responsibilities, each member has to adjust and cope with these new circumstances. Some members may adjust easily, while others may struggle to find a sense of predictability and stability. Some changes in the family system can require patience and a slow adjustment to find how to obtain a balance of functioning, while other changes can be so minor that adjusting requires little effort and attention. This example demonstrates that one factor, such as a parent starting a new job, can significantly affect the entire family system. Similarly, autism, although seemingly and previously treated as an individual disability, does not exclude the entire family system being affected in some way, shape, or form.

Families on the autism spectrum are unique because the challenges of autism are frequently changing, especially as a person moves through the stages of development. What a family might experience when their child is six may be drastically different when the child turns seven or becomes an adolescent. Families of autism experience unique stressors and difficulties

DOI: 10.4324/9781003451266-6

compared to families who have all neuro-typically developing children. Thus far, this book has focused on current research on families of autism, diversity, the Ecosystemic Structural Family Therapy (ESFT) model, early diagnosis and clinical concerns, the Autism Trait Scale, school-age years and what to expect, and finally, how to navigate school psychological assessments and Individualized Education Programs (IEPs). This chapter will highlight the importance of subsystems, such as working with siblings, provide an extensive summary of a research study that explores the sibling experience of autism through a family systems lens, and discuss clinical implications and conclusions for mental health providers and families.

Specific Focus on Subsystems

In many families, even those who do not include a member with a disability, there is often a child who presents with more difficulties and struggles with social, emotional, behavioral, or academic obstacles. In contrast, we often notice another child or children demonstrating opposite characteristics within those same families. When examining families from a family systems lens, individuals unconsciously attempt to balance one another by expressing emotions, personality traits, and behaviors. For example, if one individual is shy in the family, there is likely another person who is vocal and extroverted. Differences can go as far as mental health challenges, substance abuse, and life choices. As a result, families tend to have members who can appear drastically different, resulting in some being identified as the "problem child" or "golden child." Families of autism are not exempt from this fascinating phenomenon of homeostasis. In fact, research supports that many neurotypical (NT) siblings of autism consciously and unconsciously navigate their families by finding ways to achieve emotional stability, taking on adult-like responsibilities, being high achievers, or attempting to become small (Fontes, 2023).

Some readers may wonder how families maintain balance and adjust to one another when there is one child and two caregivers. When there is one child on the spectrum, it is common for parents to take on differing roles, which include responsibilities, emotional expression, and how each copes with challenges. For example, the parent with primary caretaking responsibilities, such as cooking, bathing, and transportation to and from school, may express more negative emotionality and feel like the "bad parent." In contrast, if the other parent supports the system in more financial ways, spending less time with the child, they may demonstrate less emotional reactivity and express healthier coping, thus resembling the "good parent." Caregivers may not continuously take on these roles, but due to lack of energy, limited resources, frustration, and work schedules, parents do what they must to keep the system functioning. In the context of this work, subsystems are defined as any person, dyad, or group within a family. All subsystems have importance, since the whole is composed of multiple subsystems; however, some subsystems will be more central in considering the psychological treatment of the family on the autism spectrum. The subsystems we propose may be most central to family therapy with this population are the parent dyad, the parent and grandparent relationship, grandparents exclusively, stepparents, and additional caretakers such as in-home support aides, and finally, the sibling subsystem.

Grandparents

Do you know anyone who was raised by their grandparents? Have your grandparents played a significant role in your life? In 2018, the US Census reported that 7.82% of children between 0 and 18 lived with a parent and a grandparent (U.S Census Bureau, 2018). An essential subsystem within the family is the relationship between the parent and their mother or father, and the relationship between the grandparent and grandchild. Families on the spectrum face unique challenges and needs compared to families that have all NT children. Families with autism may require additional financial, emotional, and structural support. Prendeville and Kinsella (2019) explored the grandparent experience in families who have a child with autism. The researchers found that grandparents recalibrate and strengthen the family system. In all family types, grandparents can bring a sense of relief. However, children with behavior challenges may especially need the calming essence that grandparents can provide. In a nationwide survey, Hillman et al. (2017) found that after obtaining the opinions from almost 2,000 grandparents, many shared their wish to connect with their grandchild, the frustrations with limited care for autism, and joy in celebrating their grandchild's progress. Although the findings may be outdated, Harris et al. (1985) conducted a remarkable study examining grandparents' experiences through a family systems lens. One finding that appeared consistent among the 43 participants was that grandparents shared a fairly optimistic view of their children and grandchildren with autism. This notion is most interesting because the grandparents also had more positive beliefs about their grandchild's difficulties with autism and the overall impact autism has on the family. For example, the parents in this study shared that since their child with autism was born, there were negative changes made to the family, whereas grandparents did not entirely agree that these changes existed or were as negative. Could this be a harmful belief or be helpful? One argument is that believing the child with autism has fewer difficulties than in reality may shift how the grandparents treat them, thus shaping a normative and typical family dynamic. In contrast, this belief could invalidate parents who may be struggling and need grandparents to see how autism truly affects the family. This phenomenon also speaks to the power of perception. Of course, parents and grandparents want to focus on the positive and believe their family is well and wonderful. However, some perceptions may have unintentional consequences. Clinicians, teachers, and mental health providers need to inform families, including grandparents who have vital roles, of the realities of autism, including family impacts, the child's abilities, and the severity of symptoms. Beyond perception, how do grandparents actually experience their grandchild? Desiningrum (2018) found a positive correlation between grandparents' role in families and the grandparents' well-being. In other words, the more active a role a grandparent plays in a family of autism, such as providing financial and emotional support, the more positively the grandparent reports their well-being. This finding is not entirely surprising when we look at Erickson's psychosocial stages of development, in which the main task in middle adulthood is to find purpose in life by creating and producing for the generations to come. Grandparents can do this through work, child-rearing, and community service (Broderick & Blewitt, 2014). Ultimately, the psychosocial task is to find purpose in life. Grandparents who can find purpose and value in supporting their families may provide positive outcomes for their well-being.

Research on Siblings of Autism through a Family Systems Lens (Fontes, 2023)

The following will describe and explore a unique study on the sibling experience of autism through a family systems lens. The researcher (Fontes, the first author of this book) utilized open-ended and semistructured questions to interview ten NT adolescents and young adults about their experience of having a sibling with autism. Interestingly, not only did Fontes gather authentic, unfiltered responses about siblings' experiences, but she took it a step further by prompting questions that explored sibling roles within the family system, paternal perceptions, differential treatment, and how autism is spoken about in the home. Using a family systems lens, the researcher obtained rich information about how families of autism manage to function and relate to one another. The researcher's findings will guide and inform the clinical implications for the remainder of this chapter.

Findings (Fontes, 2023)

Having a Brother or Sister with Autism is Complex

The researcher found that being a sibling of autism is unique and complex, and affects some members of the family. Siblings experience differential rules and expectations that their parents have for them than they see exhibited toward their autistic siblings. This study also found that NT siblings have variable beliefs about whether or not their families could manage without them. NT siblings appear to play unique roles in the family system and have significant insight into how their families adjust and function over time to meet the needs of autism and the family system. More specifically, the researcher found that siblings reported both positive and challenging aspects of having a brother or sister with autism, especially when processing how their parents respond to autism. These NT siblings often feel protective of their brother or sister with autism spectrum disorder (ASD), but can also feel resentful at times. This stark contrast in feeling both warm and cold toward one's sibling with ASD creates a unique relationship. A NT sibling must hold onto these differing feelings and figure out how to navigate the unique relationship dynamics. Most sibling relationships come with distinctive facets and possible feelings of love or frustration; however, what is unique to families of autism is that NT siblings need to make sense of their inner world when they know, at times, their brother or sister cannot always "control" how they think, feel or behave. Also suggested in this study is that siblings feel parentified. NT siblings still tend to be placed in more parental roles. One could imagine how roles and responsibilities might change within a family when they experience multiple risk factors. Last, and perhaps most interestingly, in comparison to other research studies on families of autism, Fontes found that NT siblings have difficulty expressing negative emotions and vulnerability.

A Silver Lining

A concept not often observed in the literature is the positive aspects of having a sibling with autism. However, in Fontes' study on siblings, she found that NT siblings reported that having a brother or sister with autism made them compassionate and empathetic while also improving their ability to communicate with all people, regardless of their having a disability or not. This is quite interesting because historically, there has been an assumption that having a child with autism will cause issues or difficulties in NT children. However, that is not to say that NT siblings do not experience any challenges. This study also found that NT siblings experience unique benefits that may progress children socially and emotionally, and that siblings believe that their personality structure and way of relating to others have primarily been influenced by having a sibling with ASD. Thinking back to the family system, it may be possible that NT siblings experience advanced social and emotional development. If another child in the home is having social and emotional difficulties, one often counterbalances those deficits with strengths. It is unclear what may be the cause of increased social maturity, although it appears to be a significant finding in several research studies.

Differential Treatment of Children

This study had results that suggest that NT siblings expressed that their parents treated them differently than their siblings with ASD, specifically that parents had higher expectations of NT siblings. Although some NT siblings understood why differential treatment was necessary, many expressed feeling left out or neglected. This facet is not uncommon in families of autism, where one child often receives less parental attention and care when parents intentionally or unintentionally exert their parental resources onto the child with autism. Of course, not all families with autism experience vast differences in how children are treated. Many families can manage to provide appropriate care to each child. It is important to note that many factors may influence a parent's ability to "evenly" spread attention and care to each child. For example, reasons that affect parents may be due to the level of autism a child has, how many children are in the home, whether a parent is single or partnered, whether families have access to appropriate medical and educational resources, and the parent's overall well-being. Some NT siblings expressed that their general needs and mental health were disregarded, and there was an unspoken expectation to take care of themselves. In some families with two or more children on the autism spectrum or with other disabilities, NT children often get pushed to the side, regardless of meeting parental expectations. The notion that NT children believe parents have higher expectations of them could be because it may take much more for a parent to "notice" when an NT child has demonstrated something that one would expect some praise for. NT children may attempt to get straight A's or become star athletes to obtain the affection and love from their parents they feel is missing for typical behavior such as getting a "B" on a test or scoring a point in a sports game. In contrast, some NT children may stray in the opposite direction and misbehave or distance themselves in order to cope with differential treatment or receive negative attention from caregivers. In essence, an NT child may feel that any recognition from a parent or adult is better than none.

Do Families Talk about Autism?

The researcher also found that NT siblings perceive their parents as having both positive and negative feelings about their sibling with autism, thus creating a complex experience. It is evident that siblings mostly learn about autism through various resources such as their parents, school, and social media (Fontes, 2023). NT siblings also reported that when their families spoke about autism, conversations varied in frequency but were mostly initiated when their siblings with ASD were experiencing some challenges. However, NT siblings believed parents attempted to focus on the child with autism's success. This is interesting because it brings the topic back to family systems and homeostasis. When a topic may potentially threaten the family's emotional stability, they attempt to balance the negative by shifting into positive discussions around autism. Families may also do this to promote a more positive and encouraging environment rather than fixate on all of the challenges of ASD. In some families where grandparents play a significant role, the topic of autism may not be discussed as often. As time passes, research and understanding of autism advances. Each generation may have a different belief or bias about what autism is and the best approach to treating behavioral concerns. Some grandparents may have harmful views about autism that may influence the emotional climate of the family. When there is unspoken tension, parents may avoid talking about autism with their own parents to protect themselves and their children. However, if parents avoid talking about autism, they may lack additional support they could be receiving, even if it is simply venting about a difficult day. Clinicians should include grandparents in treatment to understand what they know and need to learn more about regarding autism. Grandparents should know they can play a vital role in keeping a family strong. Of course, not all parents may want their mother or father to be part of their lives in regard to autism, and that will always be up to each family's unique circumstances, but the literature is clear that treatment including several generations has substantial positive effects.

Neurotypical Sibling Role in the Family

Fontes found that NT siblings play a significant role in the family system, especially regarding assuming varying degrees of responsibility, being the emotional homeostats, and maintaining family stability. A main takeaway of this chapter should be that NT siblings have essential roles within the family system, and it would be helpful to include siblings in family therapy. A profound finding from the sibling study is that NT siblings expressed the importance of advocating for one's mental health needs. In other words, NT siblings expressed that they had struggled to access appropriate support for their own mental and emotional well-being. Their struggles were not explicitly identified, but it is essential to acknowledge that NT siblings may want help. This finding informs clinicians, researchers, and families that NT siblings need a voice in the family. One can use their voice not only in the home but in individual or family therapy.

Now that we have a better understanding of how siblings experience autism and what it all means, how do we use this knowledge to inform the treatment of families? Many NT siblings reported that they have taken on parental roles and responsibilities, specifically at the onset of having a sibling with ASD, and feel like an older sibling regardless of sibling order. Some of these roles were self-imposed, and others shared that their parents requested for them to partake in additional responsibilities to strengthen the functioning of the family system (Fontes, 2023). Similarly, (Tomeny et al., 2017) found that NT siblings are more likely to be parentified, which is a significant finding in the autism literature. Taking on a parental role results in complex shifts in the family structure, which may lead to feelings of resentment in NT siblings. When a child or young adult has to help their parents get their sibling ready for school by assisting them to pick out their clothes, or making them a bowl of cereal, one would expect some feelings of annoyance, but most siblings would be willing to help. However, in many families with a child on the autism spectrum, NT siblings may be asked to help with changing soiled undergarments, feeding their brother or sister, or even taking on legal guardianship of their siblings. Many of these responsibilities are not typically negotiated but often delegated out of necessity to assist the family in managing day-to-day. Of course, there are NT siblings who enjoy helping and would not change a thing about the roles they play in the family. An important finding from this sibling study is that it provides insight into the push and pull between loving one's siblings and being filled with resentment.

Some readers may be reflecting on their sibling relationships and saying, well, I love my brother or sister, but they get on my nerves, too. Isn't that normal? What is different about families on the spectrum is that families with all NT children are not commonly asked to do things outside the boundaries of what is age appropriate or unexpected for a sibling relationship. Families on the spectrum tend to create a new sense of normal in that it may be standard for an NT sibling to run and grab clean underwear for his seven-year-old brother, although it is crucial to highlight the impacts this may still have on children. Although it will be discussed in a later book, some NT adults may be asked to become legal guardians of their brother or sister with autism. Asking a person who may be trying to plan the rest of their future to do this, will then create burdens of serious legal and caregiver rights. In many instances, NT adults would likely welcome the role and feel proud to be viewed as responsible and mature enough, although still, there may be complex and conflicting feelings underneath their sense of obligation. For example, an NT adult may feel honored by the request to become their sibling's legal guardian. However, they might fear how this could affect their future. It may be challenging for an NT adult to share with their family that taking on legal guardianship is terrifying, but they may feel as though they have no choice. Later in this book, we will explore the realities of adult siblings on the spectrum and how to prepare families for long-term care and support.

Overall, it appears NT siblings hold onto frustration while also expressing great care and love for their siblings with autism, thus highlighting a complex relationship. Jones et al. (2019) found that siblings who held positive perceptions of their sibling with ASD were more likely to express positive coping abilities. Fontes (2023) did not explore coping mechanisms in her sibling study; however, many of the NT siblings reported having difficulty expressing vulnerability, specifically around negative affect and emotional needs. This would lead one to believe it may be challenging to access healthier coping mechanisms if NT children or adults are less likely to communicate that they are struggling.

It is Hard to be Vulnerable

Let us take a moment to think about times when we or someone we know might have needed help but faced some obstacle in receiving that support. There may be infinite reasons that limit people from being vulnerable; this issue may help explain why NT siblings may find it challenging to share about their internal world. Interestingly, Fontes found that NT siblings shared that as they became older, their restricted emotional expression was largely maintained in various relationships, such as with romantic partners. For example, if an NT child learned that things were easier for everyone by not sharing when they were distressed, they also did this into adulthood with other relationships. In other words, if a person grew up not voicing their needs, they were less likely to use their voice in romantic relationships. In the sibling study, it appears that NT siblings adapted and learned to become "small" and reduce any additional stress for their family, thus teaching themselves to restrict emotional expression (Fontes, 2023).

Calling all Families to the Front Line

Thus far, we have focused on more of the challenging aspects that NT siblings face having a brother or sister with autism. However, one should not fear; there is hope for families on the spectrum. Another multifaceted aspect of being a sibling of autism is the lifelong journey of learning about autism, how to function within the family system, and how people relate and connect with their siblings. These findings shed light on the reality that being a family on the spectrum is a long journey demanding deeper understanding and development. Each family will have a different path and various obstacles. As the saying goes, "If you have met one person with autism, you have only met one person with autism," and families are no different. It may be the case that children can understand more complex topics through the natural maturation of child development. In other words, when children mature intellectually and emotionally, the potential to comprehend the complexity of autism improves as well. For example, young NT children may not understand why their family must leave a 4th of July parade because their sibling with autism is feeling overwhelmed and is unable to calm themselves down due to the increased sensory overload. A few years later, that same NT child may be able to understand that some people with autism have difficulty with sensory stimulation and not argue with their parents if they have to leave somewhere early. The sibling study highlights the notion that the way families adjust and grow within the context of autism has profound effects on the family system. Interestingly, Kovshoff et al. found a similar phenomenon: it is not autism in isolation that presents families with challenges but rather how they can adapt and adjust to autism as a family unit (2017). For example, a child on the spectrum named James is out with his family for a fun day at their local park. The parents sit on a bench nearby, watching their four children laugh and play together. James digs in the mulch and enjoys searching for any odd objects that get lost in playgrounds. Nearby, another child is on the swings, which begin to make a loud screeching noise as the child sways back and forth. Immediately, James cries in hysterics and balls his fits up with mulch, throwing the dirt around, regardless of who may be walking by. James' parents realize right away that he is sensitive to the noise from the swings and go to grab his noise-cancelling headphones. His older sister, Emma, attempts to soothe him by adding pressure to his shoulders and back and asking him to focus on the color of his shoes. Soon, his brother, Matt, jumps onto a tire swing that spins with vicious speed, saying, "Hey, James, come catch me, I am spinning into outer space." James is fascinated by space, enjoys spinning, and begins calming down after watching his brother twirl in circles. James joins his brother Matt, and their sister spins the boys together.

This example demonstrates the simple but very common challenges of autism and individuals being sensitive to sensory stimulation, such as particular noises. Notice that the family did not get angry with James, leave the park, or tell the other child to get off the swings. The family did not yell at James, tell him to knock it off, or become frantic, attempting to soothe James. They came prepared, responded with empathy, and knew how to help. The parents and siblings also remained calm and knew James enough to jump into action. This example also speaks to the fact that each family member knew what triggered James. In some cases, families should inquire about what might be triggering sensory overload or anxiety if the person is able to find ways to communicate what is wrong. One should not assume that all family outings will end with rainbows and butterflies. Of course, there will be times when parents, for various reasons, have limited patience, resources, support, and energy to respond to any of their children. Difficulties will arise, and some may feel like small storms that put a damper on the whole day. Similar to a storm, some will have to pass, and families should do their best to manage until the storm is over. What is most vital is how families attempt to respond to challenges rather than how challenging the obstacle may be.

My Sibling with Autism made me Who I Am

When exploring how autism affects siblings, some individuals reported that their siblings were either nonverbal or had limited abilities to communicate, which taught them the value of communication. Specifically, in Fontes' study, NT siblings spoke about gaining increased patience, empathy, and insight into how people communicate, which they practice throughout their lives. One could imagine that growing up with a brother or sister who has difficulty with communication would require additional patience and effort to relate and find ways to communicate. Siblings shared about being open-minded and often checking in with others who may be struggling, which directly reflected how individuals learn to process their relationships and understand emotional expression. Interestingly, NT siblings appear to have unique and improved skills in reading others' nonverbal cues but have difficulty expressing their own distress. One should not assume that simply because an NT sibling is empathic and mature, they would communicate when they might need additional support.

There is Still Hope

It is important to note that many siblings expressed that having a brother or sister with autism can feel like any other sibling relationship, which includes fighting, playing, wanting attention from parents, and learning from their sibling, thus resembling a typical sibling connection (Fontes, 2023). This finding is not new and was explored by Walton and Ingersoll (2015), who found that relationships of autism are no better or worse than NT sibling relationships. To further expand this idea, siblings of autism also shared that they would not change who their sibling is, but rather only their ability to communicate. It is quite wonderful to know that even when NT siblings may experience complex, difficult relationships with their brother or sister, they would not change who they are. Parents should take this into consideration if they are feeling guilt or anxiety around the obstacles NT children may face. In fact, NT children often appear to love their siblings with ease still and enjoy the relationships regardless of autism. However, the majority of participants in this study, regardless of gender identity, expressed that if they could change anything about their sibling, it would be their ability to communicate.

The Forgotten Child

NT siblings frequently believe they receive less parental attention due to their sibling with ASD needing more time and resources, which is also emphasized in Morgan's (1988) literature review that found that NT children receive less parental attention from caregivers. As mentioned earlier, this is not a new finding; however, it is important to further understand this as it relates to family systems and individual well-being. When siblings with ASD were praised for accomplishments that fell within an appropriate developmental range, NT siblings still felt they were scrutinized more for making trivial mistakes (Fontes, 2023). In many ways, this seems reasonable because in comparison to children with ASD, many NT individuals may have the ability to accomplish different skills and tasks. NT individuals may also be expected to complete certain tasks without assistance, even at an earlier age, reinforcing the expectation to be more independent. Parents of children on the autism spectrum might forget that NT children still need appropriate support and validation on typical developmental milestones. It is essential that parents are reminded of these milestones and take a step away from the unique successes of their child with ASD. For example, a parent might become elated by their five-year-old who was once nonverbal, being able to communicate in short phrases. However, for their NT 12-year-old who ran for student council and won class president, it may appear trivial in comparison. This is not to say that all parents have a skewed perception of milestones and child success, although it is important to process how families provide praise acknowledgment and find ways to make all children feel valued and seen.

What might be the most interesting about this notion of differential treatment is that although participants shared frustration about differential treatment, many understood why their parents behaved in this way, thus allowing participants to accept their reality with more empathy and compassion (Fontes, 2023). This finding is supported by (Kawal et al., 2004), who found that the perception of fairness is associated with the quality of sibling relationships. In other words, when children or adults can understand why their parents are treating them differently, it may mediate the psychological and emotional impacts of the differential treatment. For example, if an NT child knows why they do not receive a special bedtime routine, they might be able to shift their feelings of frustration and loneliness to empathy and acceptance, which reinforces (Kowal & Kramer, 1997) that when children can justify differential treatment, they have more positive experiences of their siblings with autism. For example, if a parent explains to their NT ten-year-old: "I know you want me to put you to bed and stay a little while until you fall asleep, but sometimes your sister needs mommy to help your sister relax before bed … autism can make bedtime or transitions difficult … you are so good at getting ready for bed. I know I can trust that at 9 p.m., if I walk past your room, you are already in bed with the lights off and starting to fall asleep … I am so impressed with you because you do not need my help to fall asleep … but I know you wish I could spend more time with you at bedtime; I bet you might feel a little left out … how about I come in and give you an extra hug and tuck you in after your sister is asleep, what do you think?"

This example demonstrates how a parent can be honest and open about why they do not spend additional time with their ten-year-old at bedtime compared to their sister with autism, specifically highlighting that autism itself affects how one manages the world. This example also gives the NT child empathy, validation, and a small offer of attention that may provide more warmth. Even a parent taking the time to note the difference can provide a child with emotional comfort and understanding. The mother also reframes the child's ability to get themselves ready for bed as a strength and provides praise for the child's ability to do it alone. Notice that the mother did not apologize or attempt to overaccommodate the child with an unreasonable offer. At times, apologizing can unintentionally send a message that promotes sympathy for their sibling or shift the view that "my sibling is bad or not capable" versus "my sibling has difficulty because of autism, but it does not mean they can't do things." Overapologizing may make a child feel they need to console a parent who is struggling to do it all. The goal is to make the NT child feel seen, validated, and comforted. It is also important that the parent feel as though they can follow through with their offer of additional attention and that it is realistic. For example, the parent did not say, "I am so sorry, you are such a good kid; if you can go to sleep by yourself every night, I will take you to Disney." It is important to stay away from the overuse of rewards because children may start to believe that attention and love are only contingent on "not being a bother," thus reinforcing the belief that NT children need to stay out of the way and be "perfect." It is also essential to allow NT children to ask questions and wonder about autism and how it affects their siblings. Of course, some apologies are necessary and can be soothing, for example, "I am sorry I did not know that you felt left out." This example focuses on the internal experience rather than apologizing for autism, which we know we cannot make go away.

I Need A Hug Too

Along with siblings noticing differential treatment and receiving less parental attention, they also reported needing to be more independent and perfect. Many participants in Fonte's study spoke about the lack of attention from their caregivers, which appeared to be indirectly linked to parental expectations that children should be able to do more within the home. In regard to increased independence at an earlier age and having more responsibilities than non-ASD siblings, participants perceived this experience as a need to grow up quickly and take care of themselves. The example above about the mother giving less attention to her ten-year-old speaks to an appropriate developmental task most preadolescents should be able to complete without significant support. If the ten-year-old child needed help making dinner, it would be inappropriate to ask a child to complete it independently, even if parents are busy helping the sibling on the spectrum. More importantly, NT siblings may believe they should be able to complete certain skills on their own, which may be unrealistic. NT siblings may also feel the need to take care of themselves mentally and emotionally. However, children and adults still need support for overall well-being. A mature NT child may still need a hug when they are frustrated or a treat when they accomplish their goals. A fascinating finding of the sibling study was that participants did not want their parents to have additional burdens or want to cause disruptions, which may be associated with the pressure to be a good example and demonstrate maturity. Family members often take on roles that promote homeostasis and complementarity within the family system. Bowen's family systems theory proposes that each person has an emotional inner process, which is not intentional; the purpose of this process, according to Bowen, is to reduce overall family tension. The findings of this study suggest that NT siblings may attempt to overcompensate through perceived perfectionism to balance ASD sibling challenges.

Sibling Roles in the Family System

It is no surprise that NT siblings have a unique role in the family system. Siblings experience varying levels of responsibility within the family system, ranging from helping with simple chores to taking on more serious parental/guardian roles. In Fonte's study, siblings also expressed variable beliefs on how important they are to the functioning of the family system. Some siblings expressed confidence that their families could manage without them and had no doubt that their absence would affect the family. In contrast, some siblings in Fontes' study had concerns that their families would struggle without them due to the vital role they play in their families. To orient us back into family systems, answer a few of these questions: Would your family have functioned without you? What roles did you play in your family system? Were you always helping and supporting others as the "rescuer"? Were you "a switchboard," "a lost child," "a nurturer," "a peacekeeper," or did you provide "comedic/emotional relief," or were you a high achiever, a perfectionist, like a "hero"? Some of us may have concluded we had varying roles or that our roles changed throughout our lives as the family changed. Keep this in mind as we further explore NT sibling roles in families of autism.

NT siblings felt that they maintained the function and emotional balance of the family system. Siblings achieve homeostasis by encouraging family members to communicate and keep the peace by reducing emotional tensions through providing comedic relief and helping family members communicate clear messages. Woodgate and colleagues found that parents experience feelings of isolation when having a child with autism (2008). Interestingly, in Fontes' study, siblings appeared to notice their parents' experience of isolation. This awareness influenced NT siblings' desire to take on some of the stress of raising a person with ASD by connecting their parents to a sense of social context outside of autism. In other words, the NT siblings themselves became the mechanism through which parents receive social connection (Fontes, 2023). This particular social connection is fascinating and appears to be unique because some families may feel like they are living in a perpetual childhood, even if they have adult children with ASD. Neurotypical adult siblings view this as a responsibility to connect their parents to typical adult communication and interaction, especially if they have few social experiences outside of the home. This would lead one to believe that parents should be connected to communities outside of autism, if possible, to balance their relational experiences, lessening pressure on children and promoting a more balanced parental life. It appears that NT siblings play a vital role in helping the family system maintain balance and stability, playing a much larger role than initially reported by many participants. Siblings may have shared that their families would manage fine without them due to their underlying belief that they should be small and stay out of the way, when in fact, it was observed that participants shared significant impacts on the overall functioning of families (Fontes, 2023).

Conclusion

The main takeaway from this chapter is to understand when treating a person with autism, it is essential to meet with the entire family and recognize each of the relationships within the family. The reader should also now have a deeper understanding of the unique experiences of families on the spectrum, with a sibling focus, and how to approach such families utilizing the ESFT approach.

References

Broderick, P., & Blewitt, P. (2014). *The Life Span: Human Development for Helping Professionals* (4th ed.). Harlow: Pearson Education Inc.

Desiningrum, D. R. (2018). Grandparents' roles and psychological well-being in the elderly: A correlational study in families with an autistic child. *Enfermeria Clinica, 28*, 304–309.

Fontes, B. A. (2023). *Sibling Experience of Autism: Through a Family Systems Lens* (Doctoral dissertation, Chestnut Hill College).

Harris, S. L., Handleman, J. S., & Palmer, C. (1985). Parents and grandparents view the autistic child. *Journal of Autism and Developmental Disorders, 15*(2), 127–137.

Hillman, J. L., Wentzel, M. C., & Anderson, C. M. (2017). Grandparents' experience of autism spectrum disorder: Identifying primary themes and needs. *Journal of Autism and Developmental Disorders, 47*(10), 2957–2968.

Jones, E. A., Fiani, T., Stewart, J. L., Sheikh, R., Neil, N., & Fienup, D. M. (2019). When one sibling has autism: Adjustment and sibling relationship. *Journal of Child and Family Studies, 28*(5), 1272–1282. https://doi-org.chc.idm.oclc.org/10.1007/s10826-019-01374-z

Kovshoff, H., Cebula, K., Tsai, H. W. J., & Hastings, R. P. (2017). Siblings of children with autism: the sibling's embedded systems framework. *Current Developmental Disorders Reports, 4*(2), 37–45.

Kowal, A., & Kramer, L. (1997). Children's understanding of parental differential treatment. *Child Development, 68*(1), 113–126.

Kowal, A. K., Krull, J. L., & Kramer, L. (2004). How the differential treatment of siblings is linked with parent-child relationship quality. *Journal of Family Psychology, 18*(4), 658.

Morgan, S. B. (1988). The autistic child and family functioning: A developmental-family systems perspective. *Journal of Autism and Developmental Disorders, 18*(2), 263–280.

Prendeville, P., & Kinsella, W. (2019). The role of grandparents in supporting families of children with autism spectrum disorders: A family systems approach. *Journal of Autism and Developmental Disorders, 49*(2), 738–749. https://doi-org.chc.idm.oclc.org/10.1007/s10803-018-3753-0

Tomeny, T. S., Barry, T. D., & Fair, E. C. (2017). Parentification of adult siblings of individuals with autism spectrum disorder: Distress, sibling relationship attitudes, and the role of social support. *Journal of Intellectual and Developmental Disability, 42*(4), 320–331. https://doi-org.chc.idm.oclc.org/10.3109/13668250.2016.1248376

US Census Bureau. (2018). *America's Families and Living Arrangements: 2019.* United States Census Bureau.

Walton, K. M., & Ingersoll, B. R. (2015). Psychosocial adjustment and sibling relationships in siblings of children with autism spectrum disorder: Risk and protective factors. *Journal of Autism and Developmental Disorders, 45*(9), 2764–2778. https://doi-org.chc.idm.oclc.org/10.1007/s10803-015-2440-7

Woodgate, R. L., Ateah, C., & Secco, L. (2008). Living in a world of our own: The experience of parents who have a child with autism. *Qualitative Health Research, 18*(8), 1075–1083.

7 Family Therapy with Adolescents and Clinical Concerns

Britney Fontes and Gwendolyn Edwards

"I Know How You Really Feel"

Regarding Fontes' sibling study (2023), the researcher found that parents have complex feelings about their children with autism. What is interesting about this finding is that parents did not directly say they have complex feelings about their children with autism, but these reports came from the perceptions of NT adolescents and adults. This speaks to the fascinating notion that adolescents notice their parents' beliefs, behaviors, and emotions. This finding also speaks to the reality that whether parents have complex feelings or not, siblings of autism believe this either way. Parents may be communicating information to their families that could be legitimately their experience or not even close. First, take a moment to think about your own parents. How would you answer this question if someone asked, "How does your mom or dad feel about your sibling or another member of the family?" Most people can produce a quick interpretation. However, regardless of whether our perceptions are accurate, we have beliefs about how others feel, which may influence our cognitions and behaviors. Let us keep this in mind as we further explore how families navigate how one another may feel within the family context.

"Shh, Honey, Don't Let The Children See You Cry"

Participants in the sibling study generally perceived that their parents had both positive and negative feelings about autism related to the diagnosis itself and autism challenges. Siblings perceived that their parents expressed substantial acceptance and support of their child with autism, which was evidenced through love, advocacy, and accommodations. Parents specifically expressed pride in advocating for autism by being part of organizations, participating in fundraisers, and ensuring their children had appropriate educational resources. Siblings noted that parents also demonstrated support by teaching their neurotypical (NT) children

DOI: 10.4324/9781003451266-7

about autism and connecting their children with ASD to support groups. A common theme that was consistent throughout the participants was that children and adults believe their parents are loving and accepting through action, not only through words. When someone says, "I care about you," we might be hesitant to believe them at face value, and one would likely search for times and actions that would support such a claim. NT siblings of autism notice love is expressed through behavior and not simply through words. This is important to understand within families and in terms of how they express care toward one another. Clinicians should also observe and inquire how family members express advocacy or general feelings. It appears that being an advocate and saying you are an advocate are very different things, and family members do notice this. This is important because a family might share that they are fine with autism, and love their family member, but express contradictory messages through their actions. Siblings also reported that their parents can feel frustrated and sad. What is noteworthy is that NT siblings specifically reported that parents may cry or express remorse about the life their child with ASD could have had or achieve to its full extent. One should consider the psychological impacts this may have on a family system. For example, let us imagine a family of four that consists of a mother, a father, a low-functioning child on the spectrum, and an NT sibling who is much older.

The father is sulking in the kitchen after dinner with his wife and sharing how he is now realizing he may not be able to have that "typical father-son" relationship he always dreamed of. His wife is consoling him and attempting to focus on all the beautiful aspects of their child with autism, and the NT sibling is hiding around the corner, listening to his parents have a very deep and honest conversation about parenting. The mother may feel shame and guilt that somehow she brought this onto her family and wants to become a supermom to overaccommodate her perception that she has somehow failed. The mother knows autism will not go away and begins to dedicate herself to being the most involved mother, giving everything to her family and leaving few emotional resources to herself. The father is angry at times and even resentful, often distancing himself from his son with autism, unsure of how to accept that his fantasies may never come true. This leaves the father disconnected and emotionally detached. The NT son feels sad for his parents and loves his little brother. He feels the pressure to make his family proud and be the fantasy his dad always dreamed of. The son begins to pick hobbies and interests to appease his father and seeks constant reassurance that his father is either having a good day or enjoys spending time with him.

The example above demonstrates how the experience and expression of grieving, guilt, and sadness can shift each family member to balance out the emotional tensions within the system. Families may be unaware that these changes happen or where their feelings of obligation or motivation come from. The example describes a distant father, an overinvolved mother, and a child seeking validation, all unique facets that occur within families on the spectrum.

Now let us imagine another family encounter with the same father and his own dad, who is 82 years old. The men are sitting in the backyard, reflecting on life and sharing words of wisdom. The grandfather turns to his son, "I know you have been stressed lately, but it can't be like this forever. I know your kid has some issues, but he will grow out of it." Frustrated, the father says, "But dad, that's not how autism works; he won't just grow out of it." The grandfather shakes his head and chuckles, "We did not have this sort of stuff back in my day." The father replies, "Dad, you would be surprised. Autism has been around for a long time; we are just learning more about it. There are better ways to diagnose it now." Although this interaction is short and perhaps a stereotype, it does highlight the reality that parents of autism are invalidated by their parents. This is not because grandparents mean to be harmful, but rather because of a lack of understanding and outdated understanding of disabilities. However, a short conversation can leave a father of autism feeling more disappointed and additional sadness and pressure. This pressure can then spill over into a marriage or build up until someone can find safer ways to express their emotions.

Another common experience that was also noted by participants in Fontes' sibling study is that parents can indirectly take out their frustration on the NT children. This finding was not particularly unexpected and is observed in other literature. For example, Rivers and Stoneman also found that parental stress can spill over to children in the family (2003). What is interesting about the perceptions of parents is that adolescents and young adults' experience of autism is similar. For example, siblings shared both frustration and love for their siblings in a similar light to how they believe their parents experience autism. It may be the case that mechanisms such as spillover effects and perception of parental experience can create a narrative for children on how to navigate autism within the family system. For example, if one perceives their parent as accepting of autism, it may be easier for one to interact with their sibling with love and empathy (Fontes, 2023). In contrast, if a parent is distant and frustrated with the child on the spectrum, children may take on similar narratives being demonstrated in the home.

Let's Talk About It

In the Fontes study, NT siblings also shared about how often their families spoke about autism and in what context. When families spoke about autism, it was frequently in response to how their children were doing and what autism challenges were being presented that day. Some autism challenges include meltdowns, public tantrums, difficulty with transitions, new experiences, sensory sensitivities, physical aggression, and issues within the school system or group homes (2023). Understandably, conversations about challenges were expressed through general frustration and anxiety. Participants noted that although conversations are initially introduced by ASD challenges, parents also focus on the success or small wins of their child with autism. In times of distress, parents seem to shift their attitudes from frustration to hope. Focusing on ASD wins could be a mechanism for families on the spectrum to cope with the challenging aspects of autism. For example, a mother might say at dinner,

> Today, I got a call from Jenna's teacher that she bit another kid and had a complete meltdown at snack time because another child accidentally drank from her water bottle since they have the same one … I know we are working on the biting, but I am so tired of hearing from Mrs. Jones about every time there is an issue … but I will say when Jenna came home today, she told me she needed to go number two, and that was incredible! I am so proud of her.

A Sibling Case Study Using the Ecosystemic Structural Family Systems Approach

Overview of ESTF

Ecosystemic structural family therapy (ESFT) is a systemic, strength-based, and trauma-informed family therapy model that has evolved from structural family therapy (Minuchin, 1974; Lindblad-Goldberg & Northey, 2013). ESFT was designed to address various problems that families present within the context of their relationships with significant people in their lives, social networks, and how they interact as a cohesive unit within their world. This model incorporates a trauma-informed modality that aims to recognize, understand, and empathize with the impact of trauma on the family when they have a member with autism. An ESFT therapist would look at a traumatic event that the family experienced and try to shift the goal of understanding what was happening for everyone in the family up until the crisis services had to be called. Overall, ESFT therapists explore communication, roles, rules, behavior patterns, and how one could start to de-escalate the emotional state in the home so that the system does not erupt in the future. This would be done, by also naming and processing the experience of the family, allowing each person to name emotions during and after the crisis or challenge. This evidenced-based family therapy approach is designed to help families of children who are experiencing behavioral problems and are at risk of out-of-home placement for their child with ASD.

Traditional ESFT therapists have a core belief system in which they navigate therapy, which includes the following:

- All behavior is a form of communication within a defined cultural context.
- Symptoms are due to the context of social interactions.
- Causality is circular, not linear.
- Families are evolving, and they continually regulate their internal structure, rules, and roles in response to developmental and environmental changes.
- What it looks like when a family adapts to demands made upon them within and beyond the family system.
- Family members relate to each other in patterned ways that are observable and predictable.
- Repetitive patterns created by family roles and rules evolve in a complementary fashion.
- Family members develop a comfortable level of emotional levels in relating to one another (closeness and distance relationships at different times).
- Families are hierarchically organized, which provides unwritten rules of interaction.
- Inadequate hierarchical structure and boundaries maintain symptomatic behavior.
- Family patterns are replicated in outside relationships.
- Rigid interactional patterns can restrain success.
- Change in family structure contributes to change in the behavior of individuals.
- Promoting alternative transactional patterns broadens the flexibility of individuals in the family.
- Families are their own best resource for change and success.

Clinical Case: Alexa, 15

Alexa is a 15-year-old cisgender, bisexual, white, Jewish, middle-class female living at home with her parents and her older brother. Alexa is currently in public education and has had an individualized education program since she was diagnosed with autism spectrum disorder (ASD), Level 1 when she was eight years old. She was assessed through the request of their pediatrician due to increased tantrums as a child, specific narrow interests, limited social interests, limited shared enjoyment with others, and due to her becoming overwhelmed in social situations in which she would begin to cry and rock back and forth. During the initial intake, Alexa's parents (Michael and Donna) discussed that what has brought them to seek treatment is that Alexa is "difficult" at home and seems "stubborn" regarding schoolwork. For any requests they make, it seems as though she "will do anything not to do what is asked." On top of the "stubbornness and difficulty," Alexa will get into arguments with her parents and not back down from situations such as doing small chores around the house, hygiene routines, homework, and going outside to try and play or make friends instead of playing video games all day. Both parents reported that Alexa has been experiencing sensory difficulties, including not liking to get wet, such as sweating, showering, and/or swimming in a pool. Alexa also does not like brushing her teeth and claims that it's painful for her, which then ends in an argument once her parents remind her of the "necessities" of hygiene. Her parents fear that she will not learn to do these things on her own, and they will be brushing her hair and teeth long after her teenage years. When asked about her social life, Alexa stated that it was "fine," to which her mother (Donna) quickly jumped in and stated that "it is not fine; she barely has friends that she talks to, which makes me upset because she is now in high school and is missing out on typical high school experiences; if she just had one friend over, we would stop bothering her." Donna and Michael went on to discuss that when Alexa was younger, making friends was easy because they could schedule playdates or pick her up and go to the park, and her older brother (Jeff, age 17) would have friends over and they would all play together; however, now it seems as though Alexa does not have an interest in making friends. Her parents are also concerned that there is some evidence of bullying going on at school due to Jeff's witnessing some of the girls in her grade teasing her to the point that he had to intervene. Alexa is interested in a romantic relationship but does not know how to go about looking for a relationship and dating. Donna (Mom), Michael (Dad), Jeff (older brother), and Alexa (Identified client with ASD) presented for therapy due to wanting to "be able to have a calmer, more functional home, and talk to each other like we used to." When they walk into the office, Donna and Alexa sit on the couch, with Michael closest to Donna in a chair and Jeff closest to Alexa in a chair, very much separated children versus parents.

As with other family intervention models, the first part of treatment involves creating both the foundation for treatment and the assessment of the problem. Within this early session, the therapist attempts to join and engage the family by naming emotions, validating feelings, reframing negative statements, and starting the assessment process by targeting focal areas for change to occur during the treatment process. In the first stage of ESFT, it is important to clarify concerns and treatment expectations while also beginning the process of building a therapeutic alliance with each member of the therapeutic system. The clinician partners with each family member to develop collaborative alliances, which ESFT therapists believe to be fundamental to all change efforts. Last, it is important to identify people and extrafamilial systems (aunts, uncles, grandparents, and chosen family members) that need to be part of the sessions and invite them to participate in the treatment process. As previously mentioned, this process may seem like there are a lot of people in one room, but to understand how the whole system functions, these extra individuals can really add a lot of important information to the therapy to help initiate change.

Therapist: Well, thank you all for coming in today. When I talked to Donna on the phone, who made the appointment, she was not sure if everyone could change their schedules to accommodate this time, but I am thankful you all did.

Michael: Is this going to be an every-week thing? I believe that we just wanted to help Alexa to figure out what was going on so that she could not be so difficult in the home. I mean, I want to support her, but I do not want this to be a weekly thing...

Alexa: (slouched in the chair) ... I'm not being difficult

Therapist: From the conversation that we had on the phone, it sounded like the overall functioning and emotional level is high in the home, to the point that there are arguments going on that are making it difficult for you all to talk to and relate to each other like you used to. At this point in time I feel like it is important to have everyone involved. Alexa, I heard you say that you are not difficult. Could you tell me more about how you are experiencing everything?

Alexa: Yeah, I mean they (gestures to mom and dad) get on my case about everything, like brushing my hair, showering, when I shower, how long I shower (makes a face and looks up at the ceiling in an attempt to roll her eyes). I told you (talking to mom) I don't need you breathing down my neck

Donna: Well, I cannot let you go to school with dirty, unbrushed hair. Who would be your friend then?

Alexa: Brushing my hair is not going to give me friends; I do not care how I look to others.

Therapist: Wow, so it sounds like both of you are frustrated with this situation of hygiene; it sounds like Alexa would like more independence, and Mom, it sounds like you would like to make sure that she is taking care of herself.

Donna: Yes, exactly. You know Michael and I will not be here forever, and I want to make sure that she is capable of living on her own; she needs to start doing these things now; I cannot do them for her forever, and it is simple things we have not even gotten to, how to make food or do laundry.

Jeff: You both act like she will be alone. You know I would not let her be on her own; she could always live with me, or I could live close to her

Michael: Yes, but what your mother is saying is that Alexa needs to take responsibility on her own, and that's not on you.

Therapist: Jeff, I noticed that you are saying that you are willing to look after Alexa, and from what Mom and I talked about on the phone, it sounds like you have protected her in school, too.

Jeff: Of course, I would do anything for Alexa. I mean, I feel like I have been (turns to parents), no offense, but I have been like a third parent since she was little. It is not as bad anymore, but for a while, I was always helping her with homework, making sure she remembered her lunchbox and turned in her homework. I used to even check in with her homeroom teacher before leaving school.

Therapist: Jeff, what I am hearing you say is that you care deeply for your sister and that, at times, you have taken on significant responsibilities to help your family.

Donna: (whispers to Michael) At least we have one child who goes above and beyond to do what we ask.

Jeff: (turns to mom) Yeah, and it almost breaks me trying to be perfect all the time, but that's not fair. Alexa tries her best; she may have difficulty sometimes, but I know when she is trying. I wish you would give her more credit.

Donna: Oh, honey, I know this; Alexa is a beautiful, fun, loving girl. She is just a beautifully messy, rigid (mom smiles), sometimes smelly girl.

Alexa: (buries her face into the couch) and groans.

Therapist: If I am hearing both of you correctly, it seems like you, Jeff, and your mom have slightly different perspectives on how Alexa might be doing. Jeff, I was wondering, since you are so close to your sister, if you can share what you think is the problem?

Jeff: Me? This is fun; I don't usually get to talk this much! Sure. So, I personally think Alexa is fine brushing her teeth; she doesn't like how our mom demands it, so what I really think Alexa wants to say is, "I will do it when I feel like it. Let me play my games," but instead she refuses by saying it hurts because when something hurts, you don't have to do it. I know when Alexa is in pretty bad pain or feeling sensory overload, and I have seen her maybe twice pushing toothpaste in her mouth and tongue when no one told her to ... also, Mom, no offense again, but you always drench the toothbrush in water, and it drips all over Alexa, which she hates ... maybe if you just barely wet the toothbrush, it would be less messy. I am sorry if that was a lot.

Donna: (turns to Alexa) Is that true? Does it hurt to brush your teeth, or you enjoy telling me no?

Alexa: (Ignores mom's questions and plays with Fidgets in the office)

Therapist: Jeff, thank you so much for sharing that insight. Donna, I am not certain Alexa enjoys refusing to do what you ask. I imagine that some arguments become so disruptive to the day, you would rather not get into it, but it might be that Alexa is not sure how to communicate how the sensory aspects of brushing trigger her, so what might be overwhelming, like water, is being communicated as pain, which is then demonstrated as refusal. Also, developmentally, most teenagers don't like being told what to do, even if it is good for them. Alexa saying no might be her attempt at agency and practicing boundaries. You might be viewing refusal as her being difficult, then Alexa gets further upset and pushes back more, thus making the situation escalate, which I imagine makes you and Michael angrier.

Donna: Well, when you put it that way, I guess we do get each other going, and I don't want to fight. But how else am I supposed to make sure she is taking care of herself? What am I supposed to do? Tell her she doesn't have to brush her teeth

Therapist: Well, I think there is probably a way to work up to the tasks with more empathy and compromise. Such as, "I understand that brushing your teeth can feel horrible. I wish we did not have to do extra things to stay healthy and clean, but we have to ... maybe we can find a fun way to do it; I know there are Star Wars-themed toothpastes you might like, and maybe we can use less water, so there is no dribble ... and perhaps instead of telling you, I can ask when you would like to try."

Alexa: (brings focus to the therapist) Star Wars toothpaste? That is cool. Where can I get some? Are you going to give me some?

Therapist: I do not have any here in the office, but I am sure we can google which store has them. I also wanted to suggest that someone like Jeff, who seems to understand Alexa well, show her how he brushes his teeth and ask if Alexa would like to join next to him. She can say no, but she should stand there and count how many seconds Jeff is brushing his teeth. And if Alexa watches the whole time, she can get five extra minutes of video games.

Jeff: Wait, but I know how to brush my teeth.

Therapist: Yes, of course, but the fear is that Alexa will not know how to do these things as an adult, and the first step is to at least teach her by modeling and giving her incentive to observe you. My hope is that over time, she will start to mimic you and not feel like someone is telling her what to do, which will reduce her motivation to push back. Plus, I think you are onto something with the water on her toothbrush

Alexa: (Grins wide and turns to Jeff) I will make you brush your teeth until the next day. I have all the power (raises hands to evil laugh). Muahaha.

Donna: What if she watches Jeff and never brushes her teeth?

Therapist: That is a reasonable concern, but it seems like Alexa might do better than we expect if we ease into it. I know hygiene is so important, but whenever there are additional pressures within the family and high expectations, we often feel too afraid to try, shut down, or give up quickly.

Alexa: (Turns to Mom) Yeah, I don't need you breathing down my neck; when you yell at me, I just want to shut my door in your face so you can't see me.

Michael: At times, it really feels like Alexa is being ungrateful for everything we do, and it is hurtful to her mother and I.

Alexa: (Drags her hands over her face) Dad, stop!

Michael: No (volume increasing), I am tired of how you talk to your mother, and they (gesturing to mom and the therapist) are right that we are not able to communicate in the home, and enough is enough, and if we are going to be here, we have to talk about this to fix this, because we cannot continue to argue and then you just stomp to your room and play video games when you are upset and then when we go after you to try and continue the conversation you say things like " I hate you, don't talk to me, shut up, I wish you weren't my parents" ... I am tired of it

Donna: You do come in and apologize later, but it does really hurt in the moment (turns to the therapist). I know she does not mean it.

Alexa: (Looking away) I don't mean it. I want it to stop in the moment .

Therapist: Alexa, what do you want to stop in the moment?

Alexa: They are just going to follow me until I say they are right and push me until I do what they say, and I don't think that they are always right.

Therapist: And Jeff, when this is going on, where are you?

Jeff: I am in my room until it gets loud enough like they are all yelling, and then I try to jump in. I try to calm the situation down, but usually get Alexa to back down enough so she can leave the room and then I try to play video games with her until she calms down

Therapist: So, at this point in time, it seems as though Alexa and Mom or Dad get into a disagreement about something, which then brings in the other parent until it escalates even more to a point where Jeff has to get involved and physically remove someone, most likely Alexa. Then, does the problem ever get solved or settled? (Donna and Michael look at each other)

Donna: No, we usually stop talking about it unless Alexa says something that is really hurtful, and she apologizes, but that's really it until it happens again, but it isn't always like that; sometimes we don't fight, or it's a little argument and then the big ones like every once in a while.

Jeff: More like every couple of days.

Therapist: What I am gathering is that through behaviors, we are all trying to communicate something, which has an influence on the next choice of action that feeds into emotions, coming full circle. I know that we were talking about hygiene, but it sounds like this happens with most disagreements in the family. For example, Mom and Dad, it sounds like there is a real fear there that when you are not here anymore, Alexa will not be able to take care of herself, and as parents, you want to be able to care for her and help her to become independent in some ways, but currently, the way that that is being communicated is pushing her further away from being able to do these activities, and, Alexa, it sounds like when Mom and Dad discuss things with you it gets to a point where you want it to stop and maybe even feel out of control of the conversation and the way to make this "stop," you have learned, that saying really hurtful things to Mom and Dad will stop everything at some point even if you do not mean what you say and feel bad about it after, and, Jeff, you and Alexa have a close relationship, and I am wondering if you have learned that your role in the family, if you want to have a voice, is to be protective of Alexa and the meditator of the disagreements. I am wondering what would have happened if you had not jumped in to rescue Alexa and found a different way to communicate with Mom and Dad.

Conclusion

Living in a family system with autism can require several life-changing shifts, as well as hyperfocused attention on the person with autism, while also creating rigid, circular, difficult ways of functioning and communicating. Each member of the family may be affected differently but still play a vital role within the family system. A person with autism can have varying degrees of obstacles and wonderful attributes. The goals of the ESFT therapist will address family challenges regardless of the level of autism, the trauma experienced, or the degree of conflict inside the home. Therapists should consider taking a holistic ESFT approach, examining the many facets of family functioning to manage autism and the constant adaptations families encounter. Each member of the family can provide strengths and unique insights that are necessary to explore to benefit overall family well-being. The ESFT therapist will take their time to understand the nuances of communication within the home and the triggers for the person with ASD, but also the emotions of other family members. The main takeaway from this chapter is that when treating a person with autism, it is essential to meet with the entire family and recognize each of the relationships within the family, not simply what they say but how things are communicated to one another. The reader should also now have a deeper understanding of the unique experiences of families on the spectrum, with a sibling focus, and how to approach such families utilizing the ESFT approach.

References

Fontes, B. A. (2023). *Sibling Experience of Autism: Through a Family Systems Lens* (Doctoral dissertation, Chestnut Hill College).

Liebman, R., Minuchin, S., & Baker, L. (1974). The use of structural family therapy in the treatment of intractable asthma. *American Journal of Psychiatry*, *131*(5), 535–540.

Lindblad-Goldberg, M., & Northey, W. F. (2013). Ecosystemic structural family therapy: Theoretical and clinical foundations. *Contemporary Family Therapy*, *35*, 147–160.

8 Older Adolescents and Young Adults

Developmental Needs and Services

Gwendolyn Edwards

Support for the Individual and Family and Dynamic Changes

Research shows that between 73% and 81% of adults with autism spectrum disorder (ASD) also meet the criteria for at least one current co-occurring psychiatric disorder (Mosner, 2019). Anxiety and depression are two mental health disorders that are most commonly diagnosed across the nation and can be more prevalent in individuals with autism. As a society, we have become more accepting of recognizing and understanding mental health, but there is still a long way to go. There is still room to improve, especially regarding stigma and how mental health impacts individuals and their families. When someone on the spectrum is going through significant life changes such as emotional, relational, puberty, educational, and significant milestones, and sibling changes, and navigating the overall family structure, support may be most beneficial during these periods. Individual or family therapy could be especially helpful for families navigating transformations.

Regardless of its severity, ASD poses many challenges for families. After acquiring an ASD diagnosis, as previously discussed in the early chapters of this book, parents can often have varying responses. At times, some parents may feel bereaved, feeling as though they are not sure how to proceed or do not know how best to parent and interact with their child, requiring more support than pre-diagnosis. Others may feel relieved and want to learn to understand and connect with their child in a more fulfilling way, and now they may feel as though they have to explain their child's behavior to others. Time, knowledge, and support can be powerful for a family's acceptance of the diagnosis. Parents are not the only ones who are influenced by this diagnosis, but also all family members, including neurotypical (NT) siblings, can have unique experiences with autism. Sibling relationships provide early social interaction, and due to their longevity, there are substantial opportunities for each sibling to influence the other. Some of the difficulties that families may navigate can be

DOI: 10.4324/9781003451266-8

inflexibility in adhering to routines, unpredictable behavior, personal care, relationships within the family, tantrums, and shifting from one activity to the next. These challenges will shift and transform as the individual with autism gets older. Some new dynamics include more complex friendships, puberty, academic challenges, independence, and NT sibling changes. The way in which individual family members approach and process these challenges may vary, and it is therefore important to gain a systemic view of the family framework.

One way of navigating this change within the system, especially with an NT sibling, is to understand how that sibling impacts the family system itself and specifically the individual with autism. For example, let's say that the NT sibling is older by three years than the sibling with autism, and when the NT sibling leaves home for college, the individual with autism may be a sophomore in high school. Not having their sibling at their school may be a difficult transition for the younger child. When siblings go to school together, the NT sibling's presence may be a source of comfort. For example, a person with autism may feel more comfortable engaging in social interactions with their NT sibling present. Additionally, the older sibling may have helped regulate their sibling with ASD when they were having a "meltdown" at home. The family may thus experience increased stress and see more emotional dysregulation in the absence of the NT sibling. In this instance, discussing the role of the NT sibling in therapy may be helpful, especially in predicting how things may shift when the family structure changes. Reflecting on the family system when the NT sibling moves away will highlight how family dynamics may be affected. Many families go through this typical milestone, but navigating it with the individual on the spectrum may look different. An example of opening communication within the family system is to discuss how the NT sibling is reacting to all of these changes, how they are feeling about leaving the home, and what would help this transition so that they can successfully navigate this new chapter for themselves. Due to navigating different stressors in the family, their own mental health struggles, and various changes in demand regarding support throughout the life span, NT siblings may experience fatigue. Siblings may also take up greater caregiving roles (Seymour et al., 2013; Nuttall et al., 2018; Critchley et al., 2021). It is extremely important to discuss the caregiver role in depth as when the caregivers get older (typically parents), they may possibly be unable to provide the support they were previously able to. For families with NT siblings, this can create a feeling of pressure, a feeling of responsibility, or even guilt to step up and provide and fulfill the caregiver role. Communication in a family therapy setting can be extremely helpful in breaking interactional patterns that are not helping or serving the family system.

Individual Emotional Changes

An area that is not always discussed regarding individuals on the spectrum is the reality of puberty and emotional changes during the adolescent time frame in an individual's life. Puberty can be an extra-fraught time for young people on the spectrum, specifically due to some of the features that define autism, including sensory and emotional issues, repetitive behaviors, and missing social cues and skills. Difficulties in these areas can make it hard for individuals to cope as they mature sexually and become more interested in friendships and dating. Girls who are on the spectrum may have a particularly tough time socially as they struggle to navigate the intricacies of neurotypical interactions. Females who are more in the mild or higher-functioning range of autism are also likely to be diagnosed with ASD later in life. Consequently, this occurs for them around puberty or as young adults. Research supports that boys are referred for a diagnostic assessment ten times more often than girls (Wilkinson, 2008; Lockwood Estrin et al., 2021). Autism is a social disorder, and one of the areas when assessing for diagnosis is looking at behavioral characteristics. We know that males and females can present socially different; therefore, diagnostically, ASD might look different across individuals. In the time of puberty and young adolescence, friendships can be intense; for males and females, there can be a strong desire to be liked and fit in, which can lead to the imitation of peers so that individuals on the spectrum may engage in camouflage or social masking. Many autistic individuals show a range of behaviors and strategies that help them mask some of their symptoms and mimic the behaviors of NT individuals to fit in with the community. Social camouflaging was first shown to be a characteristic of a person with autism who actively tries to disguise and compensate for their autism features in social contexts to blend in more easily (Tubio-Fungueirino et al., 2021). Camouflaging consists of complicated copying behaviors and/or masking certain personality features with an adaptive role that aids changes to different situational demands and is more prevalent on social occasions. Although the effect of camouflage is understudied, this concept has been referred to in the literature as imitation, copying, masking, and compensation. Camouflaging is increasingly receiving more attention on various social media platforms. Camouflage may impose many difficulties on autistic individuals, including depression, anxiety, and burnout due to the constant pressure of having to feel as though they have to present themselves in a particular way to be socially accepted.

If the notion of camouflaging is still unclear or unfamiliar, the following example will describe its nuances in more depth. Sarah is a 17-year-old female with a Level 1 autism diagnosis and presents as higher functioning; however, she really struggles with social nuances, which have led her not to have many friends or social interactions throughout high school. Before school in the morning, she runs through her day thinking about all the different social interactions that she will likely have during her classes and how she would respond to them without drawing attention to her autism diagnosis. This can look like trying to predict how others will respond, how she will respond to others, and remembering to stare at the spot between a person's eyes because direct eye contact overwhelms her. Other examples include not engaging in conversation between classes because she gets overly stimulated remembering to nod when others are talking so that they feel as though they are being listened to, using phrases that she knows are popular and helpful in the conversation, as well as minimizing or avoiding topics that surround her special interest of marine animals. Sarah has a really close friend named Beth, who is almost like a social mentor. This means that Sarah has copied or mimicked social behaviors that she has observed in Beth and engaged in that have been successful. Sarah decided to use some of those behaviors and phrases to achieve social success on her own. While these aspects of masking and camouflage have been successful at times for Sarah, they have also increased her anxiety regarding day-to-day interactions and making sure that she is not drawing attention to herself or her autism diagnosis.

Camouflaging may also lead to delayed diagnosis, which prevents individuals from getting appropriate care. One way to assist the individual and the family in navigating camouflaging and supporting a safe environment for a more genuine and fulfilling social experience can be initiated though social groups.

Social Skills Groups

Since autism was first described as a condition characterized by major difficulties in social interactions, these interactions have been a defining feature of individuals with ASD and identified as the single most powerful predictor of diagnostic status. The social impairments shown by individuals with ASD have considerable heterogeneity. Therefore, social skills training is an important aspect of intervention planning. There are a number of treatment methods, including social stories, peer-mediated interventions, scripts, script fading, social skills groups, and video modeling. Working with a social skills group on body language and social nuances, such as taking turns regarding conversations, can increase social awareness and provide more successful experiences for individuals on the spectrum. The social skills group can also be a great place for individuals to connect with others on the spectrum, share stories, and get feedback from peers who have had similar experiences. The group itself is a therapeutic process for these individuals to immediately practice and receive feedback on the skills that they have been working on, such as being able to practice social skills like taking turns, showing empathy, providing validation, using listening skills, engaging in collaboration, using verbal communication, reading body language, being held accountable to a like-minded peer group, using humor appropriately, and reading social cues. An important aspect of this type of group is the group facilitator, who also has to be able to praise individuals for using skills appropriately and provide immediate constructive feedback. This is unique because individuals with autism may not get constructive feedback from their NT peers in the school system or other social interactions.

This process helps to decrease the feelings of masking and camouflaging because it allows the individual to practice skills so these feelings do not become a negative or anxious thought process. Individuals can also get support from other peers who have difficulty in similar areas. For example, a member of a social skills group may share something that happened to her over the weekend, like a fight that she and her sibling got into over being able to play a video game on their gaming console. Another group member may interrupt the first member, make an inappropriate joke, or quote a line from the video game. The group facilitator's job would then be to pause the interaction that's happening, noticing and pointing out that it was inappropriate to interrupt the first person speaking, and allow the second individual to have an opportunity to correct their behavior while then encouraging the first individual to speak about how they felt when they were interrupted. The group facilitator may highlight that it was not appropriate to interject; however, maybe the humor of the joke was a way that the second individual was trying to make the first person feel better. The facilitator could note the appropriate time to use humor to help a friend feel better. The group social skills coordinator must be able to continue the process and intertwine different games or fun activities to learn and incorporate the social skills that the group members are learning during their group sessions.

Life Skills

As mentioned earlier, therapy can be extremely helpful during this time of transition for the family as well as the individual, and group therapy can be a great space for receiving social support and learning life skills. Families with individuals on the spectrum may navigate a delicate balancing act trying to support and promote independence while doing so in a safe way that is within the individual's capabilities. As the individual gets older, the need for independence may continue to grow, which can add stress to the family. Families may be unsure how to support the notion of independence. One way to support these goals could be working as a family on life skills and developing different daily living tasks that the individual may struggle with so that the person on the spectrum can feel more independent.

What are life skills? Life skills are sometimes called independent or daily living skills and can include self-care activities, cooking, money management, shopping, room organization, and transportation. These skills are learned over time, beginning at home at a very young age and developing further throughout adolescence and adulthood, and sometimes individuals may need more support and structure to encourage and grow these skills. Learning a wide range of life skills that apply to many areas of the lifespan is important for neurodevelopment and all ages. However, for those on the spectrum, these tasks may also include a focus on organizing, planning, prioritizing, and decision-making related to each life skill being taught.

How to Teach Life Skills?

A consistent theme throughout this book is that every person with autism is different; therefore, each presentation will need personalized support. When we look at what life skills would benefit the individual and the pace at which they are taught, it will vary from person to person. For example, one young adult with autism may ultimately be able to live on his or her own with very little support, while another may require support and services 24 hours a day, seven days a week. Categories related to life skills can include some of the following: health and safety; employment; peer relationships, socialization, and social communication; community participation and personal finance; transportation; and home living skills.

Life skills classes or independent living programs can be supportive environments for individuals to learn and practice these skills. These types of programs are usually led by a teacher or therapist, and occur in natural environments where the abilities that are being taught relate directly to the person and how they are going to live and use them, for example, learning meal prep, safety, and cooking skills in a kitchen, or learning laundry skills in a laundromat.

Many people on the autism spectrum work best with visual cues, which can be extremely helpful in teaching and promoting the practice of life skills. One way to practice and promote life skills is to create visual cues for that person, such as a checklist, which can break down a larger task into smaller, more manageable ones. For example, an individual who is on the spectrum may struggle with a morning routine even though the rest of their day seems to go smoothly. Breaking down and having a morning routine checklist could be helpful and include activities such as brushing teeth, getting a shower, combing their hair, getting dressed, and then going downstairs and getting ready for breakfast. Each checklist will look different for various members on the spectrum and their various levels of support and needs. It can also be helpful to talk about which areas of life skills would be more challenging regarding sensitivity to sensory difficulties, such as bristles on a toothbrush, combing their hair, or having a specific shower wash that doesn't produce a lot of suds. Having open communication with the individual's therapist who's teaching the life skills as well as what will work best in the system as the family develops can be key for success and ease of implementation.

College and Jobs

One of the next big steps for families in various households is the launching phase of preparing their children to leave the home. Individuals on the spectrum will also engage in this launching, but it will likely look different compared to their NT peers. Whether they're leaving the house to start a new job or navigating a new college campus environment, there can be a shift in the family dynamic in this time of navigating independence and supporting the individual on the spectrum.

Postsecondary education, such as college, can bring up new challenges for the family in making sure that the college will provide the correct and appropriate accommodations for those on the spectrum. Colleges are required to provide accommodations to students with disabilities; however, it is important to note that many of the accommodations that they received in high school may no longer be available at the college level of education. Even though some accommodations may not be provided to the student, bringing along any Individualized Education Program or 504 plans that the student had in high school can still be helpful. Other important documents that would be helpful at the start of this process would be clear identification and documentation of an autism diagnosis, providing the most current information regarding the diagnosis. Some colleges may prefer that the diagnosis be recent, and it's important to understand how each professional defines the diagnosis. Do they mean within the last five years or in the last four or three years? Information that would be important to have is the history of the student's medical, educational, and development strengths and areas of growth, and where the person still needs support. Last, families should gather diagnosis support, such as current treatment plans or accommodations that have previously worked for the student. It is imperative to start the accommodations process prior to admission. The beginning of this process will likely include researching the disability support services (DSS) office and learning about the process. For example, families may inquire about what is needed to obtain accommodations for each university. Individuals could also connect with current college students who utilize the DSS. Similarly, in our discussion in previous chapters, just like with private and public schools, each college is unique in terms of the level of support that it provides. While some colleges offer the bare minimum in terms of legal requirements, others will go well above and beyond what they need to provide students. Making an appointment to talk to the DSS office of each school that one might consider, could help narrow down the choices as to what would fit best for the individual and ease the family's stressors. Examples of support surrounding accommodations could include reduced course loads, priority registration, the possibility of substituting one course for another, extended testing time, and accessing notetakers (or receiving audio recordings of class).

Employment Transitions

Another avenue for independence can be employment. With an autism diagnosis, a person can also be eligible to receive services from vocational rehabilitation programs, which coordinate and provide counseling, evaluation, and job placement services for people with disabilities. Vocational rehabilitation supports individuals with disabilities in preparing to find and maintain a job that matches their skills and abilities. Eligibility is based on a person's disability and whether the disability presents obstacles to employment that can be remediated through vocational rehabilitation services. Each state has a vocational rehabilitation agency that provides employment service support to people with disabilities, including autism. Vocational rehab agencies can provide vocational assessments that lead up to the development of an Individual Plan for Employment (IPE), under which a variety of employment-related services can be provided, including training, counseling, job placement, and supported employment. In order to qualify for services, the division of vocational rehabilitation (DVR) reviews medical and educational history, as well as employment experience, to determine how the disability affects an individual's ability to be employed. This is a significant area where community and personal advocacy play an important role. For example, if a person needs to get reassessed for autism, being as specific as possible as to what that individual needs in this report could be helpful for the psychologist and in terms of how they are designing the tests that they would be using. The DVR may use this report to connect families with vocational services.

As we have previously discussed, regarding the Section 504 law and how it pertains to obtaining accommodations in a school setting, this law also protects qualified individuals from discrimination based on their disability. Section 504 applies to employers, public colleges and universities, and other organizations that receive financial assistance from any federal department or agency. For employment purposes, qualified individuals with disabilities are persons who, with reasonable accommodation, can perform the essential functions of the job for which they have applied or have been hired to perform. Under Section 504, a recipient of federal financial assistance may not, based on a disability, deny qualified individuals the opportunity to participate in or benefit from federally funded programs, services, or other benefits or deny employment opportunities for which they are otherwise entitled or qualified. Section 504 is also the same law that requires school districts to provide a free, appropriate public education to each student with a disability. While the Americans with Disabilities Act (ADA) also protects individuals, Section 504 requires organizations receiving federal funds to make their programs accessible to these individuals. Therefore, if one has an official autism diagnosis, they can seek protection and accommodations in all federally funded programs—employment, housing, community living, and so on.

After understanding all of the resources and supports that are available to an individual with autism, the next steps include preparing for the job search, application, interview, and obtaining employment. Creating a list of the person's skills, interests, and what they enjoy doing can help narrow down jobs that would fit within their interests as well as what is feasible for their schedule and location. The next step might include the family discussing transportation and the employment itself. For example, will the person have access to a car, public transportation, carpooling, and so forth? Being able to discuss any areas or problematic situations that could arise regarding transportation could be helpful in decreasing stress for everyone involved. Designing a résumé and possibly joining a social networking site such as LinkedIn, ZipRecruiter, CareerBuilder, or Indeed could be great places to start. Joining social media support groups revolving around autism and employment could be an area for exploring networking within those groups. Filling out job applications, as well as writing cover letters, can be a stressful experience for anyone, and even more so for individuals on the spectrum, and it could be a great place to ask for support from a therapist or other family members. The application and the cover letter can be the first impression an employer has, so finding ways to be authentic and presentable can be key in securing a job interview. Once an interview is secured, it can be helpful to practice interviewing skills and prepare for difficult or tricky questions that could arise, as well as practice techniques, to navigate unexpected questions or schedule changes that could be triggering for some people. Being able to have family, a support person, a therapist, or a friend ask practice interview questions and make it feel as real as possible to simulate the same environment that the interview will be conducted in, can be a great way to prepare for an interview. It can be helpful to watch videos of mock interviews on the Internet or record a practice interview to identify key areas that would be helpful to improve upon.

What Rights does a Young Adult with Autism have, and How do they Access them?

Throughout a child's life, they have access to different means of assessment or screening to allow them to receive accommodations, services, and support through the school-age years, but what happens beyond 18 years old? A lot of caregivers may dread what might happen after the school-age years because there tends not to be a lot of direction on how to access help. This section of the chapter will highlight different services that are available to individuals on the spectrum and how individuals and their caregivers can access them. It is important to note that aspects of Medicare, Social Security, and other legal aspects will be discussed in detail in Chapter 9 but will be introduced here.

The ADA prohibits discrimination and ensures equal opportunity for persons with disabilities in employment, state and local government services, public accommodations, commercial facilities, and transportation. In terms of employment, Title I of the ADA applies to public and private employers and prohibits discrimination based on disability when it comes to any aspect of employment, including hiring, firing, pay, job assignments, promotions, layoffs, training, fringe benefits, and more (Americans with Disabilities Act, 1990). The law also requires an employer to provide reasonable accommodation to an employee or applicant with a disability, unless doing so would cause significant difficulty or expense for the employer. If an individual does receive an official diagnosis, it is important to read about their rights under the ADA, especially if a caregiver feels their child has been treated unfairly or even discriminated against in the workplace. If there is a "reasonable" accommodation related to the challenges an individual experiences with autism that could support them in their job, a diagnosis may secure that accommodation. Some common accommodations include allowing individuals to join in on meetings on a video call if being in person is too overstimulating, allowing the use of headphones or sensory-specific tools, having flexibility in work hours, and so on.

Disability Agencies and Services

Contacting the developmental disability (DD) agency in one's state is suggested as a way to find out if one is eligible for services through the Medicaid waiver in their state. State and local DD services operate under various names across the country. Frequently, the funding for these services comes through Home and Community-Based Services (HCBS) waivers, which are made available through Medicaid. Medicaid can play a critical role in providing both healthcare and long-term services and supports that help meet the ongoing needs of adults with autism. The requirements for gaining access to these services vary from state to state. Contact the local or state agency to see if a person may be eligible.

Many individuals with disabilities who are unable to secure competitive employment rely on Social Security benefits for most of their income. Social Security Disability Insurance (SSDI) and Supplemental Security Income (SSI) disability programs are the largest federal programs aiding people with disabilities, both of which are administered by the Social Security Administration. These programs are only available for individuals with disabilities who meet certain medical criteria. One must have a diagnosis; some arguments may require an updated diagnosis to qualify for benefits. After acquiring the diagnosis and paperwork that one needs, it is important to schedule a consultation with a Social Security disability representative to understand the specific benefits a family is entitled to receive.

Adults with autism are often eligible for services to support them in various aspects of their lives. Services vary from state to state, but most involve a team component comprised of the individual, family members, friends, and coordinators from an agency or organization providing the service (if the individual has qualified for services through agencies). Although the information provided on services discussed below is not exhaustive by any means, it provides some basic information to help families begin to navigate programs and options.

Housing and Options

Increased well-being is associated with living in a good-quality and socially cohesive neighborhood. For individuals with autism spectrum disorder, there may be a greater emphasis on these qualities since individuals on the spectrum have difficulties with socialization and tend to get overwhelmed by sensory stimuli in the environment, among other symptoms (Ben-Sasson et al., 2009; Roux et al., 2013; Jones-Rounds et al., 2014; Stacey et al., 2018). However, housing is a rarely explored topic in autism research, even though this can be a huge area of concern for caregivers (Scheeren & Geurts, 2015). There is a worldwide trend toward deinstitutionalization; however, only a minority of autistic adults live independently (Anderson et al., 2014; Hewitt et al., 2017; Mandell, 2017). An estimated half of all autistic individuals continue to live with parents well into adulthood (Howlin & Moss, 2012). Understandably, aging parents often express deep concerns about the future and the living situation of their adult child with autism once they are no longer able to take care of and support them. It may be helpful to start this discussion by sharing realistic expectations about independent living. Some discussions may include how much support the individual needs regarding daily living tasks; what works for the individual and for the family; how to plan for emergencies; who will be available for social support; at what level, if any, NT siblings are involved in care if they want to be; and what are the goals and wishes in living independently for the individual with autism. In looking at daily living tasks, it is important to discuss what areas are aspects of a person's strengths and weaknesses. Daily living tasks are defined by Sidney Katz, et al. (1963) as bathing, dressing, toileting (getting on the toilet, using the toilet, and cleaning themself), transferring (moving in and out of bed/chairs), continence (controlling bladder and bowel function), and feeding (including meal preparation). Communicating daily living task needs is crucial in discussing an individual's and family's level of comfort regarding independent living (Katz, 1983). The discussion of these tasks can help narrow down areas of needed extra support and how that individual and family are going to address those needs. In addition, highlighting tasks can help direct the type of housing options available for that person based on their individual preferences and needs (Scheeren et al., 2022).

Housing options are often the same as for any NT individual looking for a place to live; however, how they may change or look different for an individual with autism is that achieving independent living may look different. Options may include places like a single-family stand-alone home, duplex, townhouse, condo apartment, or room rental in a home. Depending on financial resources, a family may consider renovating a basement or adding an addition to the home so that there can be a sense of independent living for the individual with autism. This allows support from the caregivers if needed. In addition, as part of the planning process, it is important to consider the best option for the individual with autism as well as the family, whether that be securing housing such as ownership, rental, lease, or co-op. Additionally, there are many different community-based residential service options. Some of these options combine housing and support services, while others allow the housing and support services to be arranged separately.

Other Types of Supportive Living

As previously discussed, what type of support an individual with autism would need to live semi-independently or fully independently will depend on the person and their needs. This section will describe the types of supportive living to aid in this decision-making process.

Supported Living offers services to individuals with disabilities who can live in a home or an apartment. The services, minimal in nature, are based on the individual's specific support needs and are provided by caregivers working under the direction of the individual. If the supports are personalized, anyone can benefit from the supported living model, including those with the most significant support needs. Supervised Living (semi-independent living) offers more direct and intensive structured support available 24 hours a day. The individual may live in a house or apartment, either alone or with others. Functional life skills such as banking, shopping, cooking, and going to doctor appointments can be taught or supported by staff.

When considering residential options, Group Home Living has been the traditional model for individuals with developmental disabilities. In a group home, several people with disabilities live together with on-site staff who are always present. Instruction at these facilities focuses on independent living skills and community activities. The house is owned and operated by a provider agency that also employs and supervises the staff.

Group Living/Ownership (Co-op) is similar in some ways to group home living, with the exception that the house itself is owned by a group of families or individuals who have formed a cooperative agreement. Caregivers are hired by the co-op and, in some cases, by an agency contracted by the co-op to provide support services.

Lastly, Assisted Living Facilities/Intermediate Care Facilities (ICF) aid with personal care and activities of daily living such as bathing, grooming, dressing, and more. In some states, ICF programs also provide medication assistance. Assisted living communities differ from nursing homes in that they don't offer complex medical services. On the other hand, nursing homes can be used to provide housing and support services to those who need more medical support care.

References

Americans with Disabilities Act of 1990, 42 U.S.C. § 12101. (1990). www.ada.gov/pubs/adastatute08.Htm

Anderson, K. A., Shattuck, P. T., Cooper, B. P., Roux, A. M., & Wagner, M. (2014). Prevalence and correlates of postsecondary residential status among young adults with an autism spectrum disorder. *Autism, 18*(5), 562–570. https://doi.org/10.1177/1362361313481860

Ben-Sasson, A., Hen, L., Fluss, R., Cermak, S. A., Engel-Yeger, B., & Gal, E. (2009). A meta-analysis of sensory modulation symptoms in individuals with autism spectrum disorders. *Journal of Autism and Developmental Disorders, 39*(1), 1–11. https://doi.org/10.1007/s10803-008-0593-3

Critchley, E., Cuadros, M., Harper, I., Smith-Howell, H., & Rogish, M. (2021). A parent-sibling dyadic interview to explore how an individual with Autism Spectrum Disorder can impact family dynamics. *Research in Developmental Disabilities, 111*, 103884. https://doi.org/10.1016/j.ridd.2021.103884

Hewitt, A. S., Stancliffe, R. J., Hall-Lande, J., Nord, D., Pettingell, S. L., Hamre, K., & Hallas-Muchow, L. (2017). Characteristics of adults with autism spectrum disorder who use residential services and supports through adult developmental disability services in the United States. *Research in Autism Spectrum Disorders, 34,* 1–9. https://doi.org/10.1016/j.rasd.2016.11.007

Howlin, P., & Moss, P. (2012). In review – Adults with autism spectrum disorders. Canadian journal of psychiatry. *Revue Canadienne de Psychiatrie, 57,* 275–283. 10.1177/070674371205700502.

Jones-Rounds, M. L., Evans, G. W., & Braubach, M. (2014). The interactive effects of housing and neighbourhood quality on psychological well-being. *Journal of Epidemiology Community Health, 68*(2), 171–175. https://doi.org/10.1136/jech-2013-202,431

Katz, S. (1983). Assessing self-maintenance: Activities of daily living, mobility, and instrumental activities of daily living. *Journal of the American Geriatrics Society, 31*(12), 721–727. https://doi.org/10.1111/j.1532-5415.1983.tb03391.x

Katz, S., Ford, A. B., Moskowitz, R. W., Jackson, B. A., & Jaffe, M. W. (1963). Studies of illness in the aged: The index of ADL, a standardized measure of biological and psychosocial function. *JAMA, 185*(12), 914–919. https://doi.org/10.1001/jama.1963.03060120024016

Lockwood Estrin, G., Milner, V., Spain, D., Happé, F., & Colvert, E. (2021). Barriers to autism spectrum disorder diagnosis for young women and girls: A systematic review. *Review Journal of Autism and Developmental Disorders, 8,* 454–470. https://doi.org/10.1007/s40489-020-00225-8

Mandell, D. S. (2017). A house is not a home: The great residential divide in autism care. *Autism, 21*(7), 810–811. https://doi.org/10.1177/1362361317722101

Mosner, M. G., Kinard, J. L., Shah, J. S., McWeeny, S., Greene, R. K., Lowery, S. C., Mazefsky, C. A., & Dichter, G. S. (2019). Rates of co-occurring psychiatric disorders in autism spectrum disorder using the mini international neuropsychiatric interview. *Journal of Autism and Developmental Disorders, 49*(9), 3819–3832. https://doi.org/10.1007/s10803-019-04090-1

Nuttall, A. K., Coberly, B. & Diesel, S. J. (2018). Childhood caregiving roles, perceptions of benefits, and future caregiving intentions among typically developing adult siblings of individuals with autism spectrum disorder. *Journal of Autism Developmental Disorder, 48,* 1199–1209. https://doi.org/10.1007/s10803-018-3464-6

Roux, A. M., Shattuck, P. T., Cooper, B. P., Anderson, K. A., Wagner, M., & Narendorf, S. C. (2013). Postsecondary employment experiences among young adults with an autism spectrum disorder. *Journal of the American Academy of Child and Adolescent Psychiatry, 52*(9), 931–939. https://doi.org/10.1016/j.jaac.2013.05.019

Scheeren, A. M., & Geurts, H. M. (2015). Research on community integration in autism spectrum disorder: Recommendations from research on psychosis. *Research in Autism Spectrum Disorders, 17,* 1–12. https://doi.org/10.1016/j.rasd.2015.05.001

Scheeren, A. M., Howlin, P., Bartels, M., Krabbendam, L., & Begeer, S. (2022). The importance of home: Satisfaction with accommodation, neighborhood, and life in adults with autism. *Autism Research, 15*(3), 519–530. https://doi.org/10.1002/aur.2653

Seymour, M., Wood, C., Giallo, R., Jellett R. (2013). Fatigue, stress and coping in mothers of children with an autism spectrum disorder. *Journal of Autism Developmental Disorder*, 43(7):1547–1554. doi: 10.1007/s10803-012-1701-y. PMID: 23124359

Stacey, T.-L., Froude, E. H., Trollor, J., & Foley, K.-R. (2018). Leisure participation and satisfaction in autistic adults and neurotypical adults. *Autism*, 23(4), 993–1004. https://doi.org/10.1177/1362361318791275

Tubio-Fungueirino, M., Cruz, S., Sampaio, A., Carracedo, A., & Fernandez-Prieto, M. (2021). Social camouflaging in females with autism Spectrum disorder: A systematic review. *Journal of Autism and Development Disorders*, 51, 2190–2199. https://doi.org/10.1007/s10803-020-04695-x

Wilkinson, L. A. (2008). Self-management for children with high-functioning autism spectrum disorders. *Intervention in School and Clinic*, 43(3), 150–157.

9 Older Adults and Family Changes

Prepare, Plan, and Have Patience

Britney Fontes and Scott Browning

The common refrain is that once one becomes a parent, they will always be a parent. Certainly, this is true. However, for some parents of autism, due to the needs of their adult children, the level of active parenting changes little, even as their child moves into adulthood and then midlife. The individual diagnosed at Level 3 of autism spectrum disorder (ASD) will be someone for whom support is a constant throughout their life. Certainly, someone diagnosed with Level 1 of ASD may have needs that demand attention; many at a higher level will be largely self-sufficient or in a consistent situation, demanding less parental attention. On occasion, the lower-functioning individual will also be in a facility or working with an agency that fully addresses that person's needs.

Being the parent (Scott Browning) of an adult man on the autism spectrum for whom the Level 2 category is his proper diagnosis, the responsibilities of day-to-day life have shifted but still take up time every day. The bigger concern is not the daily phone calls in which he needs to read us stories of his days or negotiate his activities with the agency that works with him. Those jobs are time-consuming but, for the most part, are fun. The greatest fear comes with the question, "What about when we are no longer here?" Who will coordinate the medical appointments, bank accounts, Social Security, living arrangements, and daily activities? It is fear of the future that is most concerning. It would be naive to suggest that the parent of one on the autism spectrum can assume that their child will be fully taken care of after the parents are no longer able to offer support.

Practical Issues for Adults with Autism

When a person ages, they approach natural developmental milestones, though when one has autism, these milestones may look different and affect the entire family system. When caregivers approach the beginning of a new stage, it can be accompanied by stress, fear, anxiety, guilt, excitement, or

DOI: 10.4324/9781003451266-9

even relief. Regardless of the whirlwind of emotions, families need to be prepared. One way to prepare is to be informed on what to expect, what one knows, and how to navigate inevitable stressors. Since each state has different laws, requirements, and services available for those on the spectrum, this section will generally describe relevant clinical concerns and typical challenges. First and foremost, any family that is seeking additional support and services must have a formal diagnosis for their person on the spectrum. A formal diagnosis is commonly obtained through the school, though one can get connected through their primary caregiver if they still do not have one on record. Some programs may even require an updated assessment and diagnosis. Many programs may also ask for documentation of medical history, financial records, Individualized Education Program (IEP) records, and psychiatric records if available. Some may wonder why any program would need access to financial records. In many cases, one must be eligible for services through Medicaid/Medicare. However, some families may make too much money to qualify for Medicaid/Medicare, influencing how they access support. Fortunately, there are different plans and programs available for families that depend on financial need and there are ways around this issue. One way to mitigate this stressor is to set up a separate bank account for the individual on the spectrum. A person on the spectrum who has less than 2,000 dollars in their savings can apply for Medicaid/Medicare. Additional plans that work around this may be dependent on the location one resides in, but other examples include ABLE accounts and a special needs trust. It is necessary to create a special needs trust if the individual does not have the ability to handle finances upon the passing of the parents. See Urbatock and Jones (2023)[1] for a specific discussion of the issues around a special needs trust. Typically, many law firms have someone familiar with the intricacies of such a trust, but it is worth discussing recommendations with other families needing to make these provisions for a local recommendation. A special needs trust may require consultation and support of a lawyer, which can quickly become expensive, though some states supply special defense attorneys who are experts in disabilities and services. An ABLE account is a savings account for those with disabilities and their families to assist in private funds, which can bridge them to essential benefits. To maintain an ABLE account, one cannot have more than 2,000 dollars in that account, but fortunately, this account will not affect Social Security Disability Insurance (SDSDI).

Other formal assessment tools that may be requested and useful for understanding a person's needs include but are not limited to the Vineland Adaptive Behavior Scale (ABS), Alpern-Boll Developmental Profile (LPRN BOLL), and Office of Vocational Rehabilitation (OVR) assessments. Some informal assessments that can paint a more holistic picture may include other school-aged assessments, family and friends' observations, and exploring the individual's strengths, skills, and preferences. It is not uncommon that, at this point, some families may begin to feel overwhelmed; this is normal and should be approached with sensitivity. There is a lot of "groundwork" that needs to be done before even getting approved for services, which is why, more than anything, families need to start obtaining, organizing, and documenting all information as soon as possible. The earlier families can begin gathering information and setting up their children for success, the easier it will be when the time comes, and the more quickly they can get their adult child support. Of course, many caregivers do not want to spend time thinking they will eventually pass away, though in some cases, families experience horrible tragedies, illness, and unexpected breaks within the family system before eventual death. Due to the unpredictability of life, this is all the more reason that caregivers should begin the process sooner rather than later. How soon is too soon? Professionals in the field would suggest beginning this process when the child obtains an IEP or 504 plan is the appropriate time to begin researching and exploring options. That does not mean a child needs a personal bank account at the age of eight, though parents can initiate the process of connecting to larger disability services to ensure as their child ages and reaches new milestones, they will be taken care of.

Where to Start Getting Support

A very effective and efficient method to learn about services, requirements, simple information about resources, and how to prepare for the future is to contact a local agency that provides a support coordinator. A support coordinator is a critical service that involves locating, coordinating, and monitoring needed services and supports for participants. Some supports include connecting families to community resources, building relationships with the family, advocating for individual rights, informing families of their rights, creating a behavior support plan, identifying goals, educating families on paid and unpaid services, and breaking down the benefits and risks of individuals' plans. Support coordinators also monitor, track, and ensure all needs are being met while being hands-on and meeting families and individuals face-to-face. Some coordinators will work directly with the person and act as coaches or teachers to assist them in meeting their goals, whether vocational, financial, or residential.

When one is connected to a service plan, there are often varying levels of support that provide increasing levels of reimbursement, financial allowance, one-on-one supervision, special living arrangements, and ongoing care long after parents pass away.

After all necessary documentation, approved qualifications, and assessments are completed, the team identifies the type, duration, frequency, and amount of each service needed, and the family can begin to access resources. A few avenues that families can use to obtain resources are the following: local agencies that work with individuals with disabilities, Support Coordination Organizations (SCOs), Administrative Entities (AEs), and the Department of Human Services (DHS) website, among others. It is important to note that qualifying for support and receiving services can be a lengthy and grueling process. Families need to remain patient, utilize a support coordinator, and advocate for the person on the spectrum. Advocacy is not a foreign concept to caregivers of autism, and the fight never stops. Due to the emotional, financial, and psychological challenges that inevitably weigh on families, they must start this process early and not wait until a crisis occurs. Families should also construct backup plans in case things do not go smoothly. Families need to discuss who would be responsible for taking over finances, who has access to private documents, and who may need to take in an individual until a more permanent plan is in place. It is essential that families understand that wait-lists are long and one program might not be the best fit. Families need to do their research, ask the hard questions, and involve as many trusting family members as they can. In short, creating plans is necessary, and a plan can give one peace of mind.[2]

Positive Aspects of Having a Middle-aged Adult on the Autism Spectrum

With maturity, many individuals become calmer and more controlled. Many of the adolescent rages and confusion fade, and the individual learns to accept many aspects of self. While housing, social life, and work life may not be perfect, many find a rhythm that allows a relationship between adult child and parent to grow closer. Sometimes, the individual on the autism spectrum might be able to offer physical assistance to aging parents. Most importantly, this relationship often shifts, and while the parent is still responsible for many aspects of the other's life, a deep bond exists, and that can be a gift.

Level of Functioning

The experience of the aging parent with a special needs adult child is unique to each person. However, as discussed earlier in this book, the three levels of diagnosed functionality in ASD tend to influence this process as well. Families on the autism spectrum who have an adult offspring on the spectrum who is diagnosed at the "lower" level, Level 3 in the *DSM-5*, will usually be working on finding a quality group home that can be supported through a combination of private and public funding. While the idea of a group home sounds impersonal for some people, it is often both a good and appropriate choice. Fortunately, for many at lower levels of adaptive functioning, the experience of living with peers and having supported activities is positive. There may be fewer uncertainties, which, for many, satisfy the desire for a structured existence with few surprises. In some cases, families attempt to keep adult children in the home for as long as possible; however, usually, a fear about how the future will unfold leads to some placement.

For parents with adult children diagnosed as Level 2, the role of active parenting does not end. Even when the individual is well placed in a supported apartment and has daily activities or work, the parent is often still handling appointments, offering emotional support, having visits, and often engaging in frequent communication. Many of these interactions are reasonably pleasant, but the volume of involvement can be noticeable. Finally, for the parent with a child diagnosed as Level 1, the experience is highly dependent on functional success. Fortunately, these individuals often know their diagnosis and thus understand how their interactional style fits into neurotypical society. While being Level 1 has the advantage of the individual being a more functional person, often with a job, friends, and possibly a romantic relationship, the challenges can still be burdensome. In addition, the individual at Level 1 is often challenged with the question of determining who to be candid with regarding the diagnosis. This decision can be very challenging among work colleagues, in particular.

Therapy with Middle-aged Adults on the Spectrum

The therapist looks to assist the family in adjusting. There are no uniform road maps for this process, but connecting families with good caseworkers, agencies, and community support is invariably useful. To demonstrate how the various concerns might be addressed, three brief case studies will look at families in which the individual on the autism spectrum is a middle-aged adult. The three cases will be based on the three levels of autism, and explore methods of how to assist these individuals and families clinically.

The following will provide therapeutic case examples describing common challenges and concerns that adults on the spectrum face as they age and their family systems change. To be consistent, the individuals and families described in this section will be from Chapter 3; however, those children, Kayla, Ryan, and Max, will now be described as adults. This will allow us to illustrate typical concerns across the spectrum of functioning. The first case will describe a therapy session with Kayla and her family. Below is an updated background.

Clinical Case: Kayla, 22

"Higher Functioning" – Kayla, cisgender female, age 22, IQ = 130

Kayla is a 22-year-old cisgender female who was diagnosed with autism at the age of 15 following a depressive episode that resulted in a comprehensive psychological evaluation. She began reading independently at age three, and academically, elementary school was a breeze. At the time, she was deemed gifted at age seven. She grew up with a group of friends she had known since preschool; they were all in the same playgroup organized by their parents/caregivers. In elementary school, she relied on her friends to introduce her to additional people and ultimately struggled to maintain many of these friendships. However, as she got older, she learned practical skills in keeping friends. Kayla has remained friends with two girls from middle school and speaks with them regularly through texting and video games. She also hangs out with one of the girls, named Olivia, several times a week. Kayla's family is close with Oliva and her parents. Kayla still strongly desires to be liked by others but is satisfied with having a couple of close friends.

Since Kayla has learned more about social cues and interpersonal conflict, she is better able to identify when someone may be teasing her. Kayla has had practice being teased by her brother and sister over the last several years. Her siblings are not intentionally mean but use the opportunity to help her practice reading sarcasm through some typical sibling rivalry.

Kayla is still particular about the textures of the foods she eats and has recently become vegan, reducing her aversion to meat textures and the aftertaste of dairy products. Kayla successfully completed her driver's test in high school. However, she experiences significant driving anxiety and will only drive on local roads. At the end of high school, Kayla did well on her SAT exam, attended college, earned a degree in math, and minored in foreign language studies. Kayla currently works at the local university five days a week as a math tutor and helps the administration department transition new foreign exchange students.

Kayla lives at home with her mother and now stepfather, and will often ask her family to drive her to work to avoid overwhelming morning traffic, especially if she is supposed to leave the house at 7:30 a.m. and if she is one minute late. Kayla can be very rigid and can become flustered when she does not execute tasks in a specific manner or time. Kalya's siblings find last-minute requests to drive Kayla extremely irritating. While her siblings have moved out to pursue their own lives, they complain to their mother that Kayla has too much power in the family. It is not realistic to expect her siblings, who now live 30 minutes away, to stop what they are doing to take Kayla to work.

Kayla enjoys work but feels depressed at times because she knows her friends and siblings have moved out of their parent's home and are pursuing romantic relationships, which she has identified as "the next chapter in a young adult's life." Kalya has demonstrated some interest in dating but is unsure how to relate to someone outside of her "safe topics." Kayla mentioned that there is a "handsome gentleman" who works at the university library, but she is having a difficult time knowing how to talk to him unless it is about movies or academics. Kayla is mostly independent but still relies on her parents to navigate social situations, finances, doctor appointments, conflicts with friends, anxiety meltdowns, and transportation.

Family: Mother, stepfather, older sister, age 31, older brother, age 29.

Therapist: Hello, everyone. I am so glad you could all make it. My Name is Dr. Fontes, so what brings us here today?

Mom: Thanks, I appreciate you being able to fit us in. So, I am not sure where to start.

Kayla: Well, that is easy. I want to move out and find a husband, and you won't let me. Which is quite preposterous, considering that both Eli and Jen have moved out. I am one of your children and I am an adult now; I have my own car, I graduated college, I have a degree, I am very smart, and by the way, I have friends and a job, so that means the next chapter as an adult person is to move out.

Mom: Honey, it's not that I don't want you to move out, I just don't think you are ready and I don't believe you are thinking clearly about what it requires to live on your own.

Stepfather: And the fact that she thinks she's going to find a husband, she still needs to date first. I don't want her inviting strange men over to her place that we don't even know.

Kayla: (To stepdad) You were a strange man when mother brought you home, and now you are married, so I think that it worked out quite fine.

Mom: Kayla, don't say that. I think you mean he was a stranger before you got to know him; he was not strange in the sense of weird or peculiar.

Therapist: If I may interrupt, can I ask how long Kayla has wanted to move out and, Mom, what are your biggest concerns?

Mom: Well, I guess Kayla has been talking about this for a few months now, ever since her best friend. Olivia. moved into an apartment not too far from the university where Kayla works. So one major issue is that my husband and I still take care of her finances and doctor appointments; Kayla gets overwhelmed when it comes to managing things with multiple steps that involve social interactions. Don't get me wrong, she's organized and could probably do our taxes in her sleep, but when it comes to going to the bank and writing checks or taking money out, she struggles. She also asks her dad at least three times a week to drive her to work because she is stressed by morning traffic.

Therapist: (Turns to Kayla) What do you think about what your mother said?

Kayla: She is correct; I hate morning traffic; banks, and paying bills frustrate me; and I do have a job at the university; in fact, I have two, and my best friend works from home, so I go see her on my lunch breaks. Oh, and I could do their taxes, but I assure you I would never do them in my sleep. That would be foolish.

Mom: Am I a horrible parent for not thinking she is ready? I know she is smart and has accomplished so much, but we are just worried this will be too much.

Therapist: No, of course not; you are experiencing what a lot of parents feel when their adult child on the spectrum is ready to take the next step into adulthood. I'm also hearing that Kayla has some pretty notable accomplishments but still needs some help from you two ... Guess what? That's pretty typical for young adults. (To the parents) What you are feeling is normal. It sounds like you really care about Kayla and want the best for her, but you have very valid concerns. And, Kayla, it sounds like you are mature and would like some more independence, similar to your peers. (To the parents) How have you managed to help her with some of these challenges that you've mentioned?

Mom: We manage okay; sometimes her sister, Jen, can quickly get her to work if either of us is busy, but it's a lot to ask, and I don't mind doing her banking and making appointments, but

I won't be around forever. How she can live on her own when she doesn't even buy her own groceries? I know that seems like a minor concern, but we have to consider all the details.

Therapist: I agree; there are many small things we would have to consider. It sounds like Kayla is a pretty smart young lady. I wonder how things would be if she learned how to navigate some of these things, such as practicing social scripts for the bank or following instructions for grocery shopping, or even making her drive through traffic and assisting her as a passenger? Essentially guide her through problem-solving.

Stepfather: I would be happy to help her problem-solve driving, but she has to be willing (looks at Kayla)

Kayla: How can you problem-solve something like driving when every time you drive, it's in a different circumstance?

Therapist: That's a fair question, and it's part of the problem-solving technique and skills; when one gets really good, the circumstances don't matter.

Mom: Things with our other kids were just different; we didn't need to think about how to do this while considering autism and how it might affect a new transition.

Therapist: This would be a new transition for everyone. That is why you are here today. In the next couple of months, we will process this together. There is no perfect solution, but I am here to support you through this and figure out just how much autism affects this transition.

Kayla: I know my autism makes it harder for me to do some things, but I am smart. I know I can be successful if they let me try. I can't be at home forever.

Therapist: I think you are right; you are very smart. So, let me ask you, have you thought about how you might handle the concerns your parents mentioned?

Kayla: Well, I would have to think about driving; morning traffic is atrocious but what I have not told them is that I really want to move in with my best friend, Olivia. She said it would help her with rent and we love hanging out even though she chews really loudly. Plus, my parents have known Olivia since we were kids, and Oliva lives close to where I work. In fact, I could practically walk or take a bus. To your other points, I think my mom could teach me how to go to the bank. I mean, I know where it is, but she could teach me how to write a check and pay a bill. Although I would not enjoy it, perhaps I could grocery shop; plus now that I am vegan, my parents keep buying the wrong things anyway, which is very annoying. It would be more efficient if I went anyway. I think I need more practice, instead of my mother doing everything. It is like a language; at first, it is hard, but after you study and practice speaking with people, it becomes easy.

Mom: Honey, I didn't know you wanted to live with Olivia. I thought you wanted to live alone because you say, "That's the true test of independence." I am actually open to that idea, but this is the most motivated I've heard you be about learning how to navigate money stuff and the grocery store.

Kayla: I am motivated. You know, I read that living at home with your parents makes you less attractive to the opposite sex.

Mom: Alright, Kayla, one thing at a time, honey.

Therapist: Kayla, I can tell finding a partner is important to you, but can we first concentrate on looking into this move and all it might involve? Relationships with romantic partners are challenging, especially for folks on the spectrum. I think that it is great that you hope to have a boyfriend, but I wonder if, for now we could concentrate on these daily life concerns?

Kayla: Yes, okay.

Therapist: It sounds like Kayla has put some thought into this (turns to mom). How are you feeling hearing her say this?

Any parent of an adult on the spectrum is justified in being anxious or afraid about their child's desire for independence, especially when they play vital roles in daily functioning. Therapists need to normalize this response and validate parents' fears as well as provide education about the natural developmental transitions for adults. Therapists should also express genuine feedback to adults on their hopes and fears to encourage their independence while also problem-solving real issues. Kayla is a young, mature, intelligent adult who has all the right ingredients to live with peers close by to her family. Like most young adults, regardless of being on the spectrum, they will need additional guidance and lessons about living on their own. Similar to other topics such as dating, families will experience some anxiety but should approach the subject with sensitivity and openness. What Kayla is feeling is normal and appropriate given her developmental age, and it is important that she is not shamed for wanting independence and a future love life. Kayla's family may not find all the solutions over time but talking about their real fears and hopes is a good place to start. Future sessions would likely focus on additional parental concerns, new responsibilities, how to initiate financial independence, and problem-solving hurdles as they arise.

Clinical Case: Ryan, 33

"Medium Functioning" – Ryan, cisgender male, age 33, IQ = 89

Ryan is a 33-year-old cisgender male who has a fraternal twin sister. Ryan was diagnosed with autism and attention deficit hyperactivity disorder combined presentation, when he was six years old. He did not talk in full sentences until he was four years old and struggled with fine and gross motor skills, as well as with maintaining eye contact. He was enrolled in speech and occupational therapies starting at age three, as well as early intervention services. Ryan always relied on his sister socially; he felt more comfortable playing with females rather than males due to struggling with coordination and thus not being athletic. Ever since childhood, he has struggled with falling and staying asleep, much to his parents' dismay. Ryan's IEP was initiated in the first grade, and he has made significant academic improvements with support and accommodations. Due to struggling with conversational reciprocity, especially when he is anxious, his sister often initiates conversations when in large groups with other peers. Ryan does not need his sister's help when he is with familiar individuals in small groups. Currently, Ryan and his sister talk on the phone almost every day, but he does not see her often. His sister, Emma, moved out of the house at 25 and, since finding her now fiancé, has moved halfway across the country. This was a significant emotional trigger for Ryan, although he has adjusted to seeing his sister only a few times a year. Emma feels a lot of guilt for "leaving" her brother and contemplates whether she has made the right decision.

Ryan still only drinks Poland Spring water from a particular plastic bottle. He will not eat green foods and will only use plastic utensils due to not liking how metal feels in his mouth. Although Ryan still does not like getting his hair wet, he will shower with reminders a few times a week.

Ryan was engaged in psychotherapy for almost a decade to help with emotional regulation, social cues, and conversation reciprocity. He learned how to express his emotions before he becomes too upset and will ask to use his weighted vest to calm him down. Ryan currently lives with both of his parents and helps his father do tasks around the house. He worked as a bagger at a local grocery store but quit after two months due to feeling overstimulated. Ryan's father recently suffered a serious heart attack and has been in a slow recovery for the last six weeks. Ryan's parents seem to deny the reality that they are aging. Emma is worried about what will happen to Ryan when they are gone. His sister is advocating that she become Ryan's legal guardian, though the family has not discussed these concerns together.

Father, Mother, Sister, age 33, sister's fiancé, age 30

Therapist: Good evening. I am so glad you could all make it. It's my understanding that Emma and her fiancé are visiting for a few months and were eager to get us together.

Emma: Yes, thank you, I know I briefly explained to you over the phone why I wanted to bring my family here, but I did not explicitly tell my parents (looks at parents worried).

Mom: What's going on, Em? You are starting to worry us...

Emma: What I'm worried about is you, Mom! And you, Dad. You are both getting old, and since Dad's heart attack, I can't stop thinking about what we would do if something happened to the both of you.

Dad: What do you mean? I am recovering; we are here; nothing is going to happen to us.

Emma: That's the thing; you don't think anything is going to happen, but that's not true. I know you and Mom don't like to talk about aging, but it's inevitable.

Mom: Yes, dear, we are aging, but what does that have to do with anything? Why are we here?

Emma: (looks at Ryan) and begins to cry.

Ryan: (Points to his sister) She's crying. You can breathe, Emma, in and out; do it like me (begins to rock back and forth to self-soothe)

Therapist: Before we continue, I would like everyone to take a deep breath, just like Ryan suggested; great job, Ryan. I can sense there are some difficult emotions coming up, and I want to spend time letting each of you share. Emma, I see you are crying. Is this a difficult topic to discuss with your family?

Emma: (Through tears) Yes, I just feel like we ignore the fact that Ryan needs us. If Mom and Dad aren't here, he will need me ... I am halfway across the country, and I'm overwhelmed. They need to see how serious this is.

Ryan: Where are Mom and Dad going?

Emma: They aren't going anywhere, bud ... but remember when Nanna got sick and she was really old?

Ryan: Yes, she was 89 years old and three months and two days, and she died.

Emma: Mhm, and remember how it was sad, but we talked about how all people will die one day and go to heaven with Nanna? Well, we don't know when that day will be, but Mom, Dad, and even you and I will die one day too... The older we get, the closer we get to death.

Ryan: So does that mean I will die in exactly 56 years, three months and two days?

Therapist: Unfortunately, death is not something we can predict, but what we can do is prepare for it if we know more about it. So, what your sister is saying is that your parents are getting older, just like your Nanna was getting old, and when they die one day or if they get sick, your sister is worried about who will take care of you. Does that make sense?

Ryan: Emma will take care of me; I am moving to Portland and bringing our dog, JoJo (Begins to stim with excitement)

Mom: Oh, sweetheart, don't talk like that; your father and I aren't going anywhere anytime soon.

Emma: Mom, you're doing it again!

Therapist: (To parents) It sounds like Emma has a very real and valid concern that the both of you are getting older, and maybe with the recent heart attack, life seemingly feels very uncertain. I share her concerns that we should all be discussing what will happen to Ryan when that time comes. But this is a slow process, and it's important to note that each of you will have a different emotional response to this topic. This is where we can find the space to understand where those responses come from and build connections to remind us that we are all on the same team. As horrible and sad as it can be talking about death, the more we talk about it, the better we can feel prepared and make more sound choices while simultaneously grieving when the time comes.

Mom: (Begins to tear up)

Therapist: (To mom) Is everything okay?

Mom: I'm just sad; you think you are going to be here forever, and you try to raise your kids so they will be alright when you're not here ... I just ... I guess I might have been avoiding the fact that Ryan's future is different. (Turns to Emma) I am so sorry.

Ryan's family is experiencing a very difficult and common reality for families on the spectrum. When parents get older, there is an inevitable heavy and painful unspoken energy that lingers around the topic of aging and death. In cases in which individuals on the spectrum rely significantly on parental support, it can be a daunting task to ask oneself what will happen when they are gone. The following sessions with Ryan's family would focus on processing their emotions and logistically planning the future when their parents are no longer around. In some cases, siblings or extended family members may become legal guardians for the person with autism. Clinicians should speak with families about how this can influence them as a whole and individually.

Clinical Case: Max, 26

"Low Functioning" – Max, cisgender male, age 26; IQ = 65 -ID

Max is now 26 years old. As a reminder, Max was diagnosed with autism at age three after his parents and pediatrician noticed that he would not respond to his name when called verbally, was constantly putting objects into his mouth, making humming noises, and often eloped. Currently, Max still elopes from time to time, so his father decided to place a special tracker in his shoes. Max is minimally verbal and often uses sounds and gestures to express his needs. He still enjoys watching cartoons, although his new interest is matchbox cars. Max's parents used to take him out more, but he still struggles with emotional regulation. When Max gets upset and is unable to communicate, he uses physical aggression to get out his frustrations. This has been a constant battle with Max and a continued effort to keep his emotions at ease. Max is also 6'2", which can be intimidating to anyone around when he is having a breakdown. Due to Max needing supervision and additional support while his parents are at work, he goes to a partial program three days a week. When the program is over, one of the aides will come to the house from 5 p.m. to 9 p.m., though this has become very expensive. Since Max needed full-time support, his stepmother had to quit her job and find another job requiring part-time hours so she could be home with Max on the days he did not attend the program.

Less than two years ago, Max's birth mother, Jane, whom he spent several days a week with, unexpectedly passed away. Max's mother had a special way of understanding him and knowing how to calm him down. Her death has significantly impacted the family, especially because Max's father and his stepmother are now full-time caretaking Max. In some ways, they have not had sufficient time to grieve because life "never seems to slow down." Since Max's father and stepmother have taken on additional responsibilities, their marriage has come last. This has become a point of tension for his stepmother. It has been hard to tell how Max is managing the passing of his mother, though he places his favorite Matchbox car by her picture every night.

Family: Father, Stepmother

Therapist: Hello, Richard and Susan, I am glad you were able to make it in for an appointment.

Richard: Thank you. Things are getting tense at home.

Susan: We knew that this had to happen. You have been in denial, and we need to have some type of life.

Therapist: Maybe you could catch me up.

Richard: We have been trying to find Max a home with a housemate, another severely autistic fellow, and around-the-clock aides. We have not been successful so far.

Susan: Come on, Richard. We, but "you" in particular, have done everything possible. What you are looking for does not exist. We will have to accept that what Max needs is a group home. He has fought against this, but the reality is that finding a home for two guys with around-the-clock care is just impossible if one is not a billionaire.

Richard: I promised Jane (Max's mother) I would not put him in a group home. It was one of her final wishes before she died.

Therapist: Richard, if this had not been a deathbed request, would you be so adamant about the Group Home issue?

Richard: Frankly, I agreed for the longest time, but I have to admit that at this point I am running out of hope for this alternative.

Therapist: Have you looked at any group homes? I ask since they vary quite dramatically from one another.

Susan: I have been doing research, Richard knows, and some of them look pretty darn good and a lot of the residents seem happy.

Therapist: I reviewed the evaluation of Max that you forwarded, and I do understand his level of functioning. And, in my opinion, many individuals do seem happier to be out of the home, with others with whom some relationship is possible. But, I realize we are talking about a deathbed promise, and strong personal feelings. This is not an easy decision.

Susan: I feel like I have been an amazing stepmother to Max. A lot of women would not have done what I have, but I love Richard, and I deeply care about Max. But I need us to have a life that

	is not full of aides in our home, limited freedoms, crisis, and turmoil.
Therapist:	Richard, would Jane have felt that you have made a sincere effort to keep this promise?
Richard:	Yeah, she and I were in agreement on wanting something special for Max. It is not just the promise, I mean, that is part of it, but it feels like a failure.
Therapist:	Have you spoken to any other families with individuals in Max's situation?
Richard:	Yeah, they all think I have been a superstar parent for trying to arrange this. I even bought a small house, found a potential roommate, but having consistent aides guaranteed, is just too hard to achieve. Susan, I have been doing research too. It just feels so hard to take the next step. I agree, you have been amazing in this journey with Max.
Therapist:	I want to take a moment, Richard, to highlight something really important you just said. Before, you noted that it would feel like a failure if you put Max in a Group Home and other parents have coined you a superstar for trying to go another route. How do you make sense of those two concepts?
Richard:	Well yeah, I am trying to do the right thing, and I think other parents know how hard it is to essentially find 24/7 care. I mean, what parent wants to send their kid off to a place that's not a "home"? I mean, they can call it a "home," but let's be real, it's like a nursing home for autism. I can't do that to Max; I would fail him, I would fail Jane, and I would fail myself.
Susan:	Oh, Rich, you know that's not true! You have been such an incredible father. You've loved Max unconditionally; you have always put his needs before your own. Max living in a Group Home does not make you a bad dad or a failure to any of us; it means you love Max so much that you are willing to make a hard decision to give him the best chance for success. Before you shut it down … just think, we could have some peace of mind knowing Max was being taken care of and you and I could get some sense of our life back…
Richard:	But Max is my life. As hard as it's been with all the chaos, money, aids, school support, day programs, meltdowns, and sacrifices, Max is all I know; he is part of me. How can I just let that go?
Therapist:	I can hear how much you love Max and how much he plays a part in who you are, and perhaps how you feel a sense of fulfillment and sense of agency. That being Max's father is largely your identity because it has affected so many aspects of your

life. I also get the sense that you closely associate Max's success as your own and put a lot of pressure on yourself. I think Susan is right in that you wouldn't be a failure if you decided Max should live in a group home, it is just a different way to love Max. And I want to clarify you would not be "letting Max go." He will still be your son, and you will still love him the same. You would still talk to him, see him. Group Homes welcome family support and visits.

Richard: (Becoming tearful) We lost Jane less than two years ago. Max is what keeps us all connected, I am not sure if I am ready to lose that too.

Max's family has deeply embedded beliefs about parenthood, failure, and identity. They are also still grieving the loss of Max's mother. Integrating their belief systems and the underlying emotional process with environmental changes, such as Max potentially living in a Group Home, is essential for healing and moving forward. One might be thinking, well, just tell Richard he is a good guy, and this is not about him; Max needs more support. However, we have to slow down and meet parents where they are. It would not benefit Max or his family to push any agenda or expect them to be ready for changes simply because we say so. Clinicians need to fully understand each person and what internal traumas or sensitive spots might be triggered before making big decisions. Richard's identity as a father is quite enmeshed with being close to Max and having control over his care. It is also evident that Richard finds value and assurance in being able to support Max, and perhaps Max living in a Group Home will make Richard feel like he failed at caring for his son. Not to mention, he made a promise to his deceased wife about never placing Max in a Group Home. Future sessions should address the complex layers of guilt, someone's understanding of what it means to be a parent, and their biases around adult care. A therapist should provide support and education around these natural transitions for many adults on the spectrum as well as correct any cognitive distortions. Richard may also benefit from individual sessions to process and heal from the death of Max's mom and whether the family can find another connection to her outside of Max. Richard could also benefit from exploring his identity outside of being a father to strengthen his ego and increase his support through his marriage with Susan. In this case example, one can see that the "work" is not entirely focused on Max but on the family system to strengthen and explore underlying mechanisms that may be getting in the way.

Each family will have a slightly different journey to navigate but may also find several similarities regarding logistics, their emotional responses to change, and complicated family dynamics. The sooner families can learn, obtain information, and plan for the future, the better they will be able to manage natural life changes and unexpected crises. As one can tell by now, including several essential family members in the process will provide a more cohesive and deeper understanding of the challenges each family will experience. Whether families connect with agencies, disability programs, support coordinators, or just with one another, it takes a team to raise an adult on the spectrum. No one should feel like they have to do it alone.

Notes

1 Urbatock, K. & Jones, JF. (2023). Special needs trusts, El Segunda, CA: Nolo.
2 I wish to thank Joshua Nielsen, a Support Coordinator, for providing essential information to guide this section on support.

10 Treating Families on the Spectrum

It's Not the End, It's Only the Beginning

Britney Fontes

Family Systems for Better or Worse

If you have a parent, you have a family system. If you are alone but exist in some community, you are part of a system. If you have grandparents, siblings, a chosen family, an adopted family, stepsiblings, or stepparents, you are part of a dynamic family system. Whether we like it or not, we exist in a world of systems. Systems can also extend to the community, school services, disability programs, and therapeutic supports. A system can also be viewed as a team. Teams comprise people with various strengths, skills, and weaknesses. For example, a sports team will assign a specific athlete to a position that highlights their strengths and gives them the best opportunity to support the team. Many of us forget that aside from the athletes themselves, there is an extensive network of individuals who may never step foot on the field but are equally as essential. Many professional sports teams require professionals and groups that work behind the scenes to help direct, structure, and progress the team toward success. Even when there is an injury, crisis, or unexpected turn of events, there are people who are ready to respond immediately. It is important that everyone understand their roles and responsibilities when being part of a team, as well as the direct and, more importantly, the indirect impact they have on the function of the system. How each discipline communicates and works together is equally as important as their set roles and responsibilities. If each discipline of a team believed they were the most important piece, you might expect significant conflict and chaos. If individual disciplines do not understand the limitations of their abilities and traditional responsibilities, we might see poor boundaries and high tensions. If a person does not believe they play a part in the team, they may not be aware of their areas of growth or unique strengths. Understanding the individual dynamics of "teams" like family systems encourages people to examine their impact, for better or worse. The foundations of family systems work similarly to the dynamics of sports teams. However, unlike sports,

DOI: 10.4324/9781003451266-10

once we exist within a family system, we cannot exactly take a day off. We may find new roles within the family "team," but it is something we cannot escape. This notion of being connected to our family systems may be overwhelming, but if we embrace the reality and seek to grow when people may feel hopeless or stuck, change is possible. When a person in a family is struggling with some identified disability, mental health concern, or just a bump in the road, each individual is likely to be affected. Whether one plays a small or significant role in the system, they are impacted by such issues. Systems and teams function on multidirectional mechanisms. In other words, people react and communicate back and forth, and each of those interactions can initiate a cascade of reactions. When a system or team experiences a problem, others will often respond to manage and balance out the weakness so that they can continue to move forward. This phenomenon is also referred to as coming back to homeostasis. When a family deals with consistent challenges or tension, they will continue to shift and change to bring the system back to baseline. This can be seen as problem-solving, preparation, practice, as seeking help, adding supports, changing roles, working together, and trying new plays or ideas.

Main Takeaways

As autism research grows and advances, the way we think, understand, and treat autism should evolve with it. We have to be open-minded when exploring the nuances of autism as well as how diversity and culture play a role. What we know now might even change in the next decade, and being flexible is essential in taking in information rather than becoming rigid in our beliefs. Autism is a neurodevelopmental disorder that can be observed on a spectrum of various social communication limitations, behavioral challenges, and restricted or repetitive patterns of behavior or interests and activities. Autism can impact a person and their family from the moment they are born or obtain a formal diagnosis. A family might be impacted emotionally, financially, psychologically, and structurally. It is no secret by now that there is a disproportion in ethnoracial diagnoses of autism between people who identify as Latinx and other ethnic/racial groups (Morrier et al., 2008). Our hope is that, in time, our researchers and research populations will be more representative of the ethnic identities that are often missed. We can't ignore the limitations and gaps in research, or else we limit the number of people who can be assisted and understood. The majority of this book discusses family systems, yet culture and diversity significantly influence each of our experiences of being part of a family or community. Addressing cultural differences could easily be a separate book, but one should recognize many of our beliefs, values, and family structures come from generations of family members long before we existed. Treating autism through a cultural and inclusive lens requires meeting with the entire family system. Utilizing a systems approach promotes visibility for multiple identity factors that influence a person and their family's daily experiences, especially culture and diversity. That being said, teachers, researchers, and clinicians need to be informed on the impact of diversity on the assessment and treatment of autism. It was intentional that we placed the chapter about diversity at the beginning of this book to orient readers and encourage them to use a cultural lens before proceeding. We hoped to prime readers to consider how culture will affect the specific topics of autism that are later addressed throughout the book.

As you may know by now, family therapy can go in multiple directions and include various individuals in the therapy sessions. The therapist will spend much time helping people understand one another and identify essential concerns and solutions. For some families, this might result in separation and the cutting off of negative emotional ties, increasing or improving communication; for others, it might be rewriting the entire playbook. Families of autism, like all families, may be close to or distant from one another, but the commonality is that they all face challenges. In some cases, this may be processing a divorce or separation, and for others, it might be navigating how to let go. Nonetheless, how families interact with one another and engage in communication is more important than autism itself. In using the evidence-supported approach, Ecosystemic Structural Family Therapy (ESFT), a clinician can be assured that they are conducting treatment that is likely to be valuable to the family on the autism spectrum. ESFT will address familial structures, attachments between dyads in the family, emotional tensions, generational hierarchies, and how to promote secondary change.

There are several benefits of using an ESFT therapy approach, including addressing family challenges regardless of the level of autism or degree of conflict inside the home. Therapists will do their best to examine family functioning and how each member adapts to change. Therapy should address each person in the room and allow them to share their experience, whether that be negative or positive. A trained ESFT therapist should provide nonjudgmental, collaborative, explorative communication with each person and facilitate the same between members. When meeting with families, there is typically more than meets the eye. Members must be honest and do their best to be open to the experience.

When treating a person with autism, it is essential to consider the entire family and recognize each of the relationships within the family system, especially siblings, regardless of their age. On occasion, therapy will be with everyone in the family, or at times, a few subsystems may be the only people attending treatment. When possible, we highly recommend that grandparents, stepparents, or chosen family members who impact the family should attend therapy as well.

We have provided readers with a unique and innovative way to understand how someone can be diagnosed on the spectrum of autism. The Autism Trait Scale (ATS) is a tool that assists one in creating a graphic profile of a person on the autism spectrum that genuinely highlights why they can be lower to higher functioning. This scale also allows a person to see that someone's degree of functioning is not all-or-nothing but rather a person can demonstrate relative strengths on a spectrum. Seven critical criteria that are often areas of concern are rated from effective functioning to problematic. It should be noted again that this tool is not used to diagnose a person with autism but rather to provide a visual map or guide that can help families identify where they might want to start in helping the person with autism. It is also an attempt to use a consistent model that can be applied to anyone on the spectrum. The ATS can be used with families, in the school, and other professionals who might need a quick visual aid to break down someone's areas of functioning. There is no perfect or "correct" way for families to complete the ATS, but creating it is insightful for the therapist to see where families may agree or disagree on what causes the most distress. In other words, the process of completing the ATS can be part of therapy itself. The ATS is designed to include various individuals in providing input into where someone may fall in each category. Other people include, the person with autism, teachers, doctors, and community members. This process is intended to help people on the autism spectrum see where they can improve and where they have strengths, hoping they can be proud of themselves and feel understood by others.

Whether the ATS is completed immediately after receiving a diagnosis or years later, navigating early diagnosis and clinical concerns can be stressful for the entire family system, especially for the parents. The start of a school year is an intimidating feat for anyone, let alone one who has to worry about supporting children who are neurodivergent. There are several factors that need to be considered, and many unknowns can create a spiral of anxiety. Fortunately, now that you have come to the end of this book, you as providers and families know how to advocate for a child. Advocacy will look different for each person, though this is a great place to start since many children are in school, caretakers may request an evaluation, follow through with updated 504 plans, and ensure schools understand a child's unique strengths and weaknesses. Providers can do their part by informing parents who do not know about these services and helping them communicate with schools. Parents can also bring the information they have learned from this book to school personnel and demonstrate their competency in student rights and services.

Once children are connected within the school, one might become quite familiar with the term Individualized Education Program, or IEP. We hope our advice will make the IEP process more productive and engage the school's key team members. The IEP process can be a long, complex, intricate journey that demands steady dedication, collaboration, and compassion from all stakeholders. The first step is to know how the IEP process can be initiated and how to obtain a comprehensive assessment to identify the essential goals and objectives for a person with autism. It should be noted again that by prioritizing a child-centered approach, we warrant that the IEP reflects not only academic benchmarks but also the holistic development and well-being of the student. This approach is done by cultivating open, flexible conversations with those who are part of the individual "team" or community of support. The goal is to encourage trust, respect, and collaboration between its members and to follow through with the appropriate accommodations and modifications to empower the person to reach their full potential. The IEP process can be stressful, but hopefully, after reading this book, readers will feel more confident in advocating for a person on the spectrum in a larger academic system.

As we know, a person with autism will always have autism, and advocacy does not stop in childhood. This is especially relevant when a person progresses through stages of development and will face new life challenges. These circumstances can require patience, flexibility, and advocacy, but the more we know, the better we can predict potential hurdles and face them with confidence. There is an abundance of information available for individuals to navigate adult life stages, as well as services to aid the person on the spectrum. Getting connected to community resources as early as possible is suggested, especially if a person lacks family or financial support. Several organizations solely exist to assist families in learning about what they are eligible for, what resources are available, and how to access them. This support can also extend to the individual raising the person with autism, such as support groups and how to get financial reimbursement through various government aid groups and insurance companies. As the person with autism ages, so do the people in their immediate family system. It should be noted that no one enjoys talking about death, loss, or what will happen when caregivers are no longer around. However, the sooner individuals can plan and prepare for these inevitable circumstances, the better off the family and the person on the spectrum will be. It is a short-term discomfort for long-term peace of mind.

Autism may be incredibly variable and unique, but there are several underlying themes that a majority of families have in common. This book's intention was to discuss these similarities and represent them in a genuine, comprehensive clinical breakdown that various readers can utilize to better understand autism through a family lens.

Whether one receives an autism diagnosis as a child or adult, the way it influences a person will inevitably be intertwined in most aspects of their life. This may be in a direct observable or indirect way that may not be identified from a quick glance. Autism will also affect the infamous system, which we all know now as the family or one's community. An essential purpose of this book was to instill the reality that autism does not exist on an island alone but that the island itself is built by and supported by various systems. The immediate family mostly compromises these systems, and the extended family, with whom the family identifies and associates within their community. This "island" would not exist or thrive without nurture, guidance, love, and courage. Sometimes, the island might be on fire, and other times, it may experience a hurricane or drought, but the island will still survive, being part of a larger ecosystem. Clinicians, providers, teachers, or anyone who treats autism should consider what it takes to help a person grow and learn and understand their role in the greater ecosystem. We also need to advocate for and support the very people who brought this person into the world. If you haven't learned that it is not isolated parts that matter as much as how the system functions as one, then this book has failed you. However, for those who skimmed through this book, we will remind you one last time. Autism should be treated by understanding its system, the family, and the very things that keep the "island" alive. Autism is an individual diagnosis, but it affects the entire family. Thus, it should be treated with the same consideration. It is not autism itself that is inherently problematic or negative. How individuals relate to one another, communicate, understand, and support the system is a better predictor for overall family satisfaction and cohesion. Families are often stronger together than apart, and working together takes time and effort. Some may think it might be easier if fewer people are involved; at times, this may be true. We all know someone who won't change no matter how much time and treatment are provided. However, families should still explore how that one person may affect the overall balance and function of the family, thus indirectly affecting the person on the spectrum. In some cases, even being a single parent may be a seemingly normal experience, though raising a person on the spectrum alone can consequently produce additional emotional fatigue, financial burden, and stress. In other words, even one caregiver and a child are a system and are connected to larger systems. Even if a family decides not to seek therapy or attempt to widen their circle of support, parents should still recognize how they still might need a breather. We might encounter individuals who will not admit they need a breather or ask for help. Someone reading this book may fall into this category. The first place to start is taking a step back and questioning what is getting in the way, what underlying beliefs one has about asking for help, and how one's family relationships make life better or worse. Can one continue to get by without making any changes? Will the person on the spectrum be set up with the most potential for success? Some people will be resistant, hesitant, and unsettled when talking about autism or will refuse to acknowledge that it even exists. Whether we meet this person in a school, a provider's office, a therapy session, a family dinner, a social gathering, or even a random outing with a stranger, the least we can do is encourage them to be open to learning more. They do not have to accept the information right away, but we can advocate for the importance of being open and flexible and giving it a chance.

If a person in the system disagrees with the diagnosis of autism, for example, a parent, grandparent, or teacher, tensions may rise. It is not uncommon that someone will not acknowledge the diagnosis, believe it exists, or will genuinely believe a person will "grow out of it." Interacting with these people can be quite infuriating. Sometimes, no matter how much research you present to them or evidence you wave in front of their face, they still may not accept the diagnosis. There are many reasons why someone may reject an autism diagnosis. Some may not have enough psychoeducation about what autism is, how it affects someone, and that it does not come and go like a cold. Some people may be unable to integrate a label or diagnosis into their ideologies due to religious or cultural beliefs. Some may have grown up in generations in which autism was not "a thing," so they thought, and so it becomes difficult to change their core beliefs about the world. Of course, some individuals are certain they "know" more than others, and so because their idea of autism does not match what is in front of them, they will reject anything outside of their schema. Finally, some may feel embarrassment, shame, frustration, confusion, or may be simply more concerned about being stubborn. Regardless of why someone might not accept or acknowledge the diagnosis, we can go back to the playbook and choose another approach that better fits the challenge at hand. Just like a team, we take a time-out, reassess and problem-solve. The play that might be more effective is to let go of the diagnosis entirely. Trying to force a diagnosis on a person will only create more tension and rigidity. We need to meet these individuals where they are. This may mean letting go of any diagnosis. Instead, we focus on the symptoms! A wise person once said that we can find control in letting go. There is nothing worse than a power struggle between headstrong individuals. From my experience, families with autism can be incredibly strong people. It might not be easy, and letting go may require being the bigger person or feeling like you've lost, but it will be more productive in the end. So, how does one talk about autism without calling it autism? Typically, when one is seeking additional support, they are meeting with teachers, mental health or occupational therapists, physicians, disability services, or community providers. What initiates this process is not typically the label of autism itself. There are often symptoms, behaviors, or challenges a person might experience. When one presents information, they don't say, "We need help with autism." Families typically say, we struggle with routines, meltdowns, rigidity, emotional regulation, feeding, dressing, behaviors, and so forth. When meeting with people who do not accept the autism diagnosis, one should speak to them in the same way. For example, instead of saying, "Well, Dad, he has autism, so he doesn't know better; you need to be more patient with him," before an argument erupts between a mother and her father, one can say, "Peter can be sensitive and gets upset easily when it comes to transitions, so we need to give him more time to self-regulate before we expect him to be ready to leave." Although this may not be a perfect science, this approach can be effective for many families. If a person is still hostile, invalidating, or ignorant, the family may need to return to the drawing board. This could mean reducing the time the person with autism spends around this family member, their overall ties, and reliance on their support, and creating a shift in the family hierarchy or boundaries. I say this to note that although we believe everyone should be given a chance, we are not prescribing this be done at any cost. Families, in fact, should set boundaries, and each one will have unique thresholds at which they will not tolerate certain behaviors or attitudes.

What About Other Diagnoses?

Autism itself can present many challenges and incredible attributes. However, what seems to bring families the most stress and difficulty is when they lack the proper information and support. This book is a great place to start for families and providers to understand how logistic and clinical concerns can be addressed together, and highlights the very common challenges families with autism will encounter. When reading this book, it would not be surprising if you considered how other individuals and their struggles may influence the family system. For example, when any individual requires significant attention and resources, many previously discussed concepts can be applied and are likely relevant. For example, many people with Down syndrome or other developmental or neurocognitive disorders may share similar phenomena with families on the spectrum. We would go so far as to say that readers who have family members with serious mental illness or severe substance abuse disorders may relate to the underlying family systems concepts broken down in this book. To be clear, we are not suggesting that having autism is similar to someone who struggles with addiction. Rather, we are saying that when someone in a family system requires additional support and inevitably affects another, the notions of communication, emotional tensions, traumas, structural hierarchies, flexibility, and attachments are more alike than different. This is only the beginning of understanding family systems and how we address clinical concerns when there is an "identified patient."

That being said, we should also consider how these other facets could affect a family of autism. For example, it is not too far-fetched to assume autism may not be the only challenge a family experiences. Due to the genetic component of autism and the emotional burdens it can impose on a family, therapists need to cover various facets of mental health and diagnosis. For example, a family with autism may also include another child with developmental delays, attention deficit hyperactivity disorder, eating disorders, anxiety, or depression. A family with autism may also comprise a mother with a drinking problem, a father with bipolar disorder, or a terminally ill grandparent. This notion reinforces the fact that all family members, if possible, should be included in family therapy. Regardless of whether a therapist is an expert in ESFT, most therapists, regardless of theoretical orientation, should consider treating other diagnoses or challenges based on a similar approach. For example, if a family member has a serious mental illness such as schizophrenia, borderline personality disorder, or bipolar disorder, therapists should inquire about how the family is functioning while supporting the needs of that individual. Does the family have emotional trauma or tensions, are siblings parentified, do parents feel burned out, shame, anger, fear, or have they simply given up? Do families agree about what the person needs the most? Do members have role confusion? Does this person need daily supervision? Is the family on the same page, or do members disagree about how to treat this person? As you can see, there are several factors that the system must consider that greatly affect the overall well-being of a family, similar to that of autism. For readers who are part of a family of autism, we realize you may not have access to an ESFT therapist. However, the next best option is finding a well-respected family therapist. Generally, any family therapy is better than none. If therapy is not an option, this book is still the right place to start, and if you have come this far, then you are already doing the work.

Selling Hope

During one's lifetime, a person will go through endless transitions and milestones. Many of us can note milestones as the "traditional" markers in life, such as graduation, getting a first job, marriage, starting a family, or becoming a grandparent, to name a few. When we think about milestones, we don't often imagine what those markers could look like or how they may not even exist for those who are neurodivergent. Until a person or couple has a child and receives that diagnosis of autism, people rarely think about what life may be like if their child/children were diagnosed with any "disability." I use that word lightly because, it is not experienced as such for many. The diagnosis of autism can be about more than simply putting a foreign label on a person but rather about potentially shifting the trajectory of an entire family's journey, from the direction the journey may take to how they may get there, which hurdles they may need to overcome, and which wonders they will find along the way. When someone begins the journey of parenthood, they are not supposed to have all the answers. Parents may even seek advice from family and friends, but most people are just as lost as the next person. After reading this book, some may still have questions, hundreds of "what ifs," and inquiries about individual circumstances. Although that is the thing, each family, each person, and each expression of autism is enveloped by endless contextual factors that make no single experience the same as anyone else. This book does not have all the answers, and it never intended to. Otherwise, we would be selling a false narrative. What we can sell is hope. We can share that with knowledge and preparation, education about supports, and resources, individuals can at least feel some sense of hope.

Reference

Morrier, M. J., Hess, K. L., & Heflin, L. J. (2008). Ethnic disproportionality in students with autism spectrum disorders. *Multicultural Education, 16*(1), 31–38.

Index